Secrets

of a

Skinny Chef

Secrets
of a
Skinny Chef

100 Decadent
Guilt-Free Recipes

JENNIFER ISERLOH
Introduction by JOY BAUER, MS, RD, CDN

RODALE

© 2010 by Jennifer Iserloh

All rights reserved. No part of this publication may be reproduced
or transmitted in any form or by any means, electronic or mechanical, including
photocopying, recording, or any other information storage and retrieval system,
without the written permission of the publisher.

Rodale books may be purchased for business or promotional use or for special sales.
For information, please write to:
Special Markets Department, Rodale Inc., 733 Third Avenue, New York, NY 10017

Printed in the United States of America
Rodale Inc. makes every effort to use acid-free ♾, recycled paper ♻.

Book design by Christina Gaugler
Illustrations by Diana Ponce

Library of Congress Cataloging-in-Publication Data is on file with the publisher.
ISBN-10 1–60529–588–4 paperback
ISBN-13 978–1–60529–588–6 paperback

Distributed to the trade by Macmillan
2 4 6 8 10 9 7 5 3 1   paperback

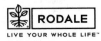

RODALE
LIVE YOUR WHOLE LIFE™

We inspire and enable people to improve their lives and the world around them
For more of our products visit **rodalestore.com** or call 800-848-4735

To Granny

CONTENTS

ix   **INTRODUCTION**

xi   **ACKNOWLEDGMENTS**

xv   **DITCH THE DIETS AND ENJOY FOOD AGAIN**

xxvii **THE PERFECT PLATE**

1   BREAKFAST

25   SOUPS, APPETIZERS, AND SNACKS

49   MAIN COURSES

101 SIDE DISHES

129 DESSERTS

163 **SKINNY SHOPPING LIST**

167 **RECIPE INDEX BY CATEGORY**

175 **NO MESS, STRESS-FREE MEALS & SNACKS**

180 **HOW TO USE LEFTOVERS**

186 **ONLINE RESOURCES**

188 **INDEX**

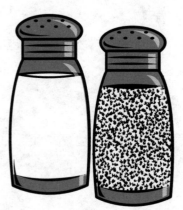

INTRODUCTION

I met Jennifer three years ago, when she helped develop recipes for my book, *Joy Bauer's Food Cures*. Since then, she has become my go-to culinary connoisseur, as well as a dear friend. Jennifer has always been extraordinarily generous with her time and expertise, so when she asked me to write the introduction for this book, I jumped at the chance to give back a little.

Truth be told, I also knew how easy it would be to gush about her recipes, because I've sampled Jennifer's creations on many occasions. I will always remember the time she showed up on a Friday night that found me too beat to stand, much less cook dinner for my family. She arrived like a modern-day Mary Poppins—calm, cool, and with a tote full of food—and proceeded to whip up her mouthwatering Stuffed Chicken Parmesan (page 66). My husband's exact words were, "No way is this healthy!" and my kids showed their appreciation by literally licking their plates clean!

As a nutritionist and avid home cook, I know how difficult it can be to prepare meals that are healthy, low-cal, and delicious. Too often, diet cookbooks sacrifice taste for results, which means they end up in a box somewhere far from the kitchen. The brilliance of *Secrets of a Skinny Chef* is that neither your waistline nor your taste buds suffer. Jennifer is a talented chef who once struggled with her own weight, and her Skinny Secrets were born of lots of trial and error. Only those that satisfied her discerning palate ended up on these pages.

Getting comfortable in the kitchen is one of the most powerful steps toward weight loss that you can take; it allows you to be in charge of ingredients and portions. It's also more economical than eating out all the time, and if you have children, it sets a great example.

So if you're really serious about losing weight and achieving your over-all health goals, I cannot recommend *Secrets of a Skinny Chef* more highly. It is imbued with Jennifer's wonderful spirit, taste, and knowledge— and I, for one, can't wait to discover more of her secrets.

Joy Bauer
MS, RD, CDN

ACKNOWLEDGMENTS

The special people in my life are the most important things to me, even more so than my enjoyment and passion for food. I think that's why my life is so rich, because I combine both my loves in what I do.

I am especially grateful to Patricia Gold, my adorable and clever granny, who raised me. She is incredibly creative, funny, and practical. She taught me the nuances of good home-cooked food while educating me about human nature while enjoying life every day by being positive and sharing with others.

Infinite, deep, and everlasting thanks to my dad and stepmom, two artists who taught me how important it is to be generous, an important quality for any home cook! Even though I'm all grown up, I still love to have their handholding and parental support.

I have two "Joys" in my life, and their name says it all. Joy Bauer, my nutrition fairy godmother, has been an endless source of support and advice. I'm not the only life she has touched and uplifted—she is changing the way we eat and live by mentoring thousands of people to live happier and healthier lives through sound nutrition. My second Joy, Joy Tutela of David Black Agency—who watched over me like a guardian angel—has an incredibly sharp eye, wit, and business savvy. She has guided me through the world of publishing with a kind and steady hand. Words cannot express my gratitude.

Thanks to the entire crew at Rodale Inc., whose enthusiasm, support, and dedication have fueled my excitement for this book. Special thanks to my editor, Shannon Welch, for her valuable suggestions and all the editing and tasting along the way, and for everything she has done behind the scenes.

I am also grateful to Marianne Hayden for honing and broadcasting the Skinny Chef mission and for helping me to become a better communicator. Special thanks to Kimberly Yorio and Caitlin Friedland of YC Media Public Relations and Yelena Gitlin of Rodale for helping me spread the word that good health and delicious meals are attainable.

A big "thank you, girl" to each and every one of my tribe of trusted female advisors: Stephanie Lyness, Jessica Seinfeld, Glenora Blackshire, Donna Mahanna, Inger Slade, Omnika Thompson, Natacha Arnoult, Susan Marks, and Leslie Dantchik have always been there with their career advice about cooking, television, and videoworks. They have guided me to become a strong, secure, and competent business woman.

Wonderful editors have taught me much about writing, and so I want to express my appreciation to the crew at *Self* magazine, especially Lucy Danziger, Carla Levy, Erin Hobday, and Tula Karras; to Kristen Dollard at Rodale; to Kat Kinsman at AOL Slashfood; and to Maridel Reyes of Vital Juice.

I also want to thank my TV friends and energetic hosts who continue to inspire: Montel Williams and the people at Montel Media; Audra Lowe along with Ashley Diamond at Better TV; Tony Tantillo; and Richard Schwartz.

A million thanks to the dozens of New York City chefs who have allowed me to train in their kitchens, starting with my chef mentor Scott Bryan, who taught me that great food is made with lots of soul and hardcore technique. Thanks to Dan Barber, Tyler Florence, and Shea Gallante for letting me see inside their worlds and being so generous with tips and ideas that only top chefs know.

Hugs to my Hoboken gang on Park Avenue and Washington Street, who taste-tested just about every recipe in the book and gave honest feedback sprinkled with loving encouragement.

And last but never least, to Uli, business partner, loving husband, and the rock that anchors me in life and everything I do. I love you, Coco!

DITCH THE DIETS AND ENJOY FOOD AGAIN

In my years as a private chef, many people have told me they're confused about nutrition, sick of dieting, and tired of putting energy into exercise programs they hate.

So why can't we stop eating fast food, consuming huge portions, and overloading on sugar? And why do we find ourselves eating even when we're not hungry?

I have fallen into the food traps myself. As a teenager, I would stop by a convenience store every afternoon to pick up my daily candy bar and high-sugar soda. Every night after dinner I'd sit and watch TV, feeling sorry for myself and thinking about how fat I looked and uncomfortable I felt.

Then one day, I gave up that candy bar and the soda! I didn't change anything else in my life—I just wanted to see what would happen if I made a minor change to my routine.

A few months later (and a dress size smaller), I understood how much that little afternoon "treat" was affecting my body. This realization became the first of many secrets that I learned on my way to becoming a professionally trained chef and recognized healthy cooking expert.

Back in my childhood, I didn't know any better. People would offer advice, vague things like "Eat lots of fruit and vegetables," "Limit sweets," and "Exercise often." But until you apply the principles to your own life, you'll never know how you can improve—and how quickly the change might come.

That's why I decided to put all my hard-won secrets into one book so that you too can focus on celebrating food and enjoying your favorite meals without feeling guilty or facing negative consequences.

Growing Up in Granny's Kitchen

I grew up in a family of food fanatics, outstanding cooks, and passionate, overindulging eaters. Granny raised me the old-fashioned way, especially when it came to food. Sit-down meals were served at regular times, and everything was made from scratch. Granny did not approve of fast food, but there was nothing wrong with having an extra serving of her home-made stew.

Granny started cooking when she was 8 years old, around the time her mother died. It was after the Depression, and with four brothers to feed and a father who worked long hours in a steel mill in Pittsburgh, she was on her own to cook for a family of six. There was none of this premade, fast-food, or frozen dinner business, so she taught herself to cook simply by doing it.

As a kid, I spent hours in her kitchen internalizing her mantras: Home-made is always the best, good food is a luxury, never skip a meal, and always clean your plate. Eating was a pleasure for her, but it was also a status symbol. We always offered guests food when they came to visit because, during the Depression, that might have been the only square meal they would have all day. The more food in your belly, the better.

Our family is Hungarian—pass the sour cream, please. And don't forget mounds of meat, piles of potatoes, and slices of hearty peasant bread. Don't waste a crumb; bread is for dipping into sauces with fresh dill and paprika-spiked stews.

Ah, yes, I remember Granny's goulash: Moist, tender bits of beef suffocated under the weight of a clinging dark red sauce. And sweets? Envision homemade pastries swirled with nuts and stuffed with spiced, buttered apples, or snacks layered thickly with sweet poppyseed paste or cooked prunes, black and glistening as melted tar.

Granny also swapped recipes with her girlfriends from the neighborhood, her Italian and Polish friends. Weekly, she clipped out ideas from the *Pittsburgh Post-Gazette* and even re-created dishes she had tasted in restaurants. She always had something new cooking on the stove.

Growing up in Granny's kitchen, it was impossible not to fall in love with food, and we overindulged. As a teen and young adult, I had weight problems. On top of eating too much "good" food, I was also a candyholic. In the mood for a treat? Well, my dad conveniently filled a drawer with loose change from his pockets, and I could help myself to candy money anytime I wanted.

When I was old enough to ride my bike to the local convenience store, I'd hit the change drawer pretty hard, grabbing enough money for a candy bar, a cake, and a soda to wash it all down. Talk about substance abuse!

I lived in a family in which everyone was overweight or obese, and I just accepted it as a matter of fact. The weight didn't matter much when I was a preteen, but as I started to notice boys, sweets took on a whole other meaning. I really had it all at age 13—pimples, braces, and 15 extra pounds buttoned into a pair of too-tight corduroys.

I noticed that all my slender friends were asked to dance while I sat on the bleachers all night. I knew something was wrong, but every night at dinnertime, that knowledge did not keep me from reuniting with my one true love: food. I felt doomed.

"Don't worry, there will be plenty of time for boys," Granny said when I complained about going to the prom solo.

I soon had my own off-campus apartment with a kitchenette where I could prepare my own meals. Too shy to go on dates, I hosted small dinner parties at my apartment, inviting a mixed crowd of fellow students, many of whom had never had weight issues. Watching and learning, I monitored myself and remedied many of my bad eating habits with simple solutions.

After college, several dress sizes smaller, I realized that food had become my greatest pleasure and my worst enemy. Food was drama. It has always held center stage in my life, and yet I had never considered mastering it by turning my obsession with food into a career.

When I finally decided to become a chef, I made the announcement to my family. Granny said, "That's great, honey." My dad said, "Why did I spend the money to put you through school if you just want to take out garbage for the rest of your life?"

In part he was right. I did start my culinary career taking out garbage as an intern in the best restaurants in New York City. It was inspiring and terrifying. I worked over 2 years on and off in many professional kitchens, without pay. Often I was the only woman, working side by side with men who did not want me there. But it was worth it. I learned from awesomely talented chefs who taught me things because they knew that I loved food as much as they did. And after a while, they accepted me into their group.

In the end, however, the one thing that made me really different as a chef was that I did not have a large, protruding belly. I was too busy eating up every culinary tip and technique. That's when the "Skinny Chef" was born. As I chopped and stirred, my follow cooks would shout over my shoulder, "Don't you know, you can never trust a skinny chef!"

With my arsenal of cooking skills, I knew that I could be the healthy, fit person I'd always wanted to be and still enjoy food. I was not the only one who wanted to live this way. In my first job as a private chef, I began to test hundreds of healthy recipes on my clients. With enthusiasm and lots of hard work, I converted my one client into many, and I figured out how to make simple food swaps and nutritious additions to transform calorie-laden comfort food into healthy favorites that stay true to what Granny knew best: There's nothing like a homemade meal.

Along the way, I worked with award-winning cookbook authors to master the ins and outs of writing recipes for the home cook, and I learned to distill a chef's experience into a simple, healthy, yet tasty one-pager— a recipe that anyone can make. The recipes in this book are the sum of my experiences, and now they are yours to enjoy!

My Six Top Secrets

Maintaining a healthy weight, or getting to that healthy weight, is not about dieting. Rather, it is about celebrating food, about eating the foods that you already love but making them a little or a lot healthier, based on how you eat now.

For many people, dieting is about deprivation; they starve themselves and eat foods that they don't really like—all in a short-term effort to lose a few pounds. Eventually, they get tired of their dieting efforts, fall off the wagon, and regain the pounds just as quickly as they lost them.

What if you could still eat the foods you love but not have to constantly struggle with looking and feeling great?

In a nutshell, it all boils down to this: Use healthy recipes; make small, manageable changes; and cook delicious, tasty meals at home for yourself as much as possible.

That's it. Really.

If you want to know a little more, here are my six principles for healthy eating!

1. Veg Out, V Is for Vitality—Add Vegetables to Every Dish

Everyone knows that vegetables are important for health, but so few Americans crave vegetables. Even those who do love their vegetables might have a hard time finding them: So much fast food and processed food doesn't contain a shred of veggie goodness.

Adding vegetables to every meal (including breakfast) isn't hard. Vegetables are grate—er, great! If you don't have a grater already, purchase an inexpensive one and grate fresh vegetables into your home-cooked meals. Even if you do decide to do takeout, add a grated carrot or a handful of spinach to the prepackaged meal.

The more vegetables you eat, the more you'll find that your tastes will change—and you'll start to crave veggies. Trust me.

Also, don't "typecast" your vegetables or their uses in meals. Here's what I mean by that:

Everyone thinks lettuce has to go in tacos, or mac and cheese doesn't have veggies. But who says so? Why not top your tacos with chopped baby spinach that is absolutely bursting with vitamins compared to iceberg lettuce? Go ahead and put some peas or cauliflower in your mac and cheese!

Adding vegetables to a dish makes it a complete meal, because they provide vital vitamins, nutrients, and fiber—yet pack few calories. And that's why vegetables are my number-one secret weapon for maintaining a healthy weight and for striking a good balance in my overall diet.

2. Fat and Fads—Learn about Fat and Avoid Dieting Fads

People get very confused about fat: Should they avoid it? Should they just ignore it altogether? I'm not saying you should be afraid of fat; you just need to know how much you're consuming each day and what kind of fat to avoid. The reason is this: Fat is calorie dense, so it's easy to sabotage your diet if you don't pay attention to fat amounts in your food.

The average American eats four to eight times more fat each and every day than their recommended daily allowance, as established by the US Food and Drug Administration. Figuring out fat isn't that hard. The normal recommended range is usually around 50 to 70 grams per day, depending on your age, activity level, and resting metabolism.

Visit the Web site MyPyramid.gov (www.mypyramid.gov) and take 5 minutes to recalibrate your mind. To put it in perspective, just one of those fast-food double-beef burgers with the fixings and the side of large fries pack about 58 grams of fat—and that's in just one meal!

Once you know the general amounts, eating the right kind of fat is important too. All you need to remember is to remove trans fats and limit your intake of *saturated* fat. Saturated fat is the kind that stays solid at room temperature, such as butter, bacon fat, and full-fat cheese.

Many clinical studies over the past 40 years have established that arteriosclerosis and heart disease are primarily brought on by an overconsumption of saturated fats as well as an *under*consumption of omega-3 monounsaturated fatty acids that you can find in foods like ground flaxseed, fish, and walnuts.

Now that you know a little bit about fat, you can start spotting dieting fads and "health trends" that might not be that healthy. Everyone knows that diet pills can be harmful to your health, and there are plenty of other health fads that can tax your heart and your waistline. Learn about them.

3. It's OK to Crave Carbs—Be a Whole Lot Less Hungry with Whole Grains

My third principle is to add whole grains whenever possible and to know how many carbs (in the form of grains) you should have per day.

When you learn your fat facts at MyPyramid.gov, you'll also discover your daily grain/bread/pasta allotment. Note the emphasis on whole grains. Unlike white processed grains, whole grains have a lot more of the minerals, fiber, and nutrients that your body needs for everything from immunity boosting to protection against heart disease.

Whole-grain carbs help you to feel fuller longer because they are high in fiber, which not only helps your heart and digestive system but also reduces hunger pangs caused by spikes and drops in blood sugar. How does that work?

Foods high in whole grain fiber and complex carbohydrates expand in your stomach, while simultaneously slowing the absorption of food sugars into the bloodstream. Both of these actions result in a more balanced blood sugar level and keep you from having those ravenous snack attacks spurred by low blood sugar levels.

So work up an appetite for whole grains—in the form of whole grain bread, pasta, and rice. You'll be amazed at how much choice is available in the carb department!

4. Be Perfect with Portions—Get Your Eyes Examined

Unfortunately, many American restaurants have skewed our perception of what makes a good-size meal—a prime reason for recent legislation in New York City calling for chain restaurants to provide nutritional information on their menus.

Readjusting your portion sizes will enable you to readjust your belt! It can be one of the easiest ways to lose or maintain weight, because for most people, the lack of balance between eating and exercise is the predominant source of their excessive weight.

Remember my experience with the daily candy bar and soda? Once you realize the impact of portion size, of eating just a *little too much* for your current activity level, you'll have secret number 4 working for you round the clock, year in and year out.

But I'm still hungry! you think. Ah, you've hit on the key point that so many diet plans fail to address. Sure, by ruthlessly eliminating many or all fat-based calories, many diets are able to quickly bring down people's weight as a direct consequence of not dealing with the high-calorie density of fats. But fats are also important in signaling satiety to the brain, so that your brain understands that your stomach is happy and full. While it's probably wise to aim for a reduced level of fats in what you eat, you should not eliminate fats entirely. The trick is to get the right amount of fat to avoid weight gain yet still keep your body metabolizing food and absorbing vitamin and nutrients.

While you might be a little hungrier at first, scaling down your portion size and increasing your intake of whole grain fiber (remember secret 3?) will smoothly transition you into a new, healthier lifestyle.

Guess what? Your appetite will readjust pretty quickly! Meaning you'll be eating the perfect portion for a healthier weight, you'll be saving more cash, and you'll be taking fewer resources from the earth to grow and manufacture your meals.

5. Look before You Eat—Lose Weight by Reading the Nutrition Label

My fifth top secret is so easy to implement, yet many people have never spent a second in their life reading the nutritional labels found on nearly every food item these days.

It's the little box titled "Nutrition Facts" that you find on the back of product packaging. It tells you what constitutes a serving size and details the amounts of fat, protein, and carbohydrates associated with a single serving.

Once you know your fat facts and calories per day, you'll look at labels with fresh eyes; it will be like taking a blindfold off! Chances are you'll start to reshelve a lot of those unhealthy prepackaged foods that used to be staples in your grocery basket.

Look at calories and fat and then check out the number of servings. If the label on a packet of crackers says 100 calories per serving, you may think that doesn't sound bad, right? But if you look at the servings line, there might be 2.5 servings in the packet, meaning you're getting 250 calories in that package of crackers!

With just a little math in the grocery aisle, you'll find it a lot easier to maintain your healthy weight.

6. Drink Up—Think about What You Drink, Be Cool with Water

I used to be a soda-holic. Once I stopped drinking soda, which amounted to 200 to 400 calories a day, I saw a real change in my weight.

But only when I took the final step to ditch diet soda for water did I see a huge improvement in my skin. What I found out, confirmed by many fashion models, is this: Most people are notoriously underhydrated, which directly affects the complexion.

Consuming appropriate levels of water enables your body to release toxins (through urine), and good hydration impacts many other functions in your body that affect the color, quality, and softness of your skin.

And there is a secret benefit to drinking water!

Some people, myself included, mistake hunger for thirst. This could mean that you're overeating 200 to 300 calories a day because you're not hydrating yourself properly. The answer is simple—start the morning with a tall, cool glass of water and continue to drink throughout the day. It could mean shedding inches off your waistline . . . or getting rid of acne.

Your Journey to a Healthier You

Once you apply these secrets in your daily life, you'll realize that the recipe for health is so easy! As the Skinny Chef, I never focus on specific diets or memorizing calories. Eating well is so much easier than that. Just remember this simple idea: *Think before you eat.*

By learning about smart and delicious meal choices (think fat content, portion size, freshness, and nutritional labels), it becomes surprisingly simple to make effortless lifestyle changes that work for *everyone, every time.* And unlike other dieting regimens, my secrets let you eat your cake and enjoy it, too!

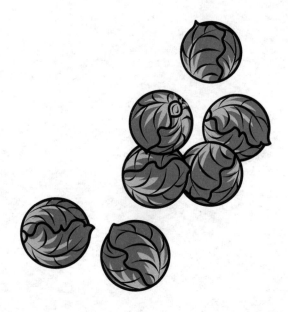

THE PERFECT PLATE

Portion size is one of the most misunderstood concepts in nutrition. Most people think of one portion as a lot larger than what the US Department of Agriculture recommends. But once you know the approximate size of a serving, it's easy to eyeball portion size. How big is ½ cup? It's about as big as a baseball or half a medium coffee cup. Once you've digested that, no one can pull the wool over your eyes when it comes to portion size, including when you read labels.

Here's a little saying, a way to remember to eat from all the food groups: Get the perfect volume of food daily.

Get—grains
Perfect—protein
Volume—vegetables
Food—fruit
Daily—dairy

Eat within 2,000 calories a day. That number might be higher or lower, depending on your age, your height, how physically active you are, and if you're a woman or man. Go to MyPyramid.gov to determine your ideal intake.

How can you stay within the calorie limits or go lower? Add more grated, steamed, chopped vegetables! They are naturally low in calories.

This is what the USDA recommends that we eat each day:

VEGETABLES: 3 OR MORE SERVINGS
Example: ½ cup veggies, like ½ cup steamed broccoli

FRUITS: 2 OR MORE SERVINGS
Examples: 1 medium apple; ½ cup chopped fruit

GRAINS: 6 OR MORE SERVINGS

Examples: 1 slice of bread; ½ cup cooked grains like quinoa

LEAN PROTEIN: 2 OR 3 SERVINGS

Examples: 2 ounces of cooked meat like chicken; 1 cup beans

DAIRY: 2 OR 3 SERVINGS

Examples: 1 cup fat-free milk or low-fat yogurt

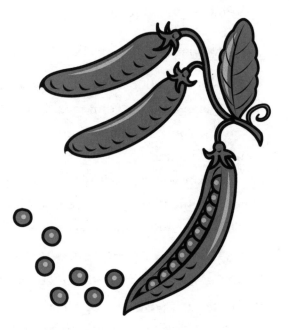

Breakfast

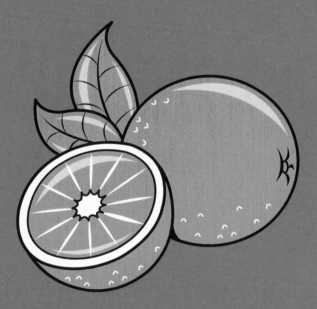

3 BACON, EGG, AND CHEESE SANDWICH

4 BACON SAUSAGE OMELET WITH ONIONS AND PEPPERS

6 BAKED EGGS AND HAM

7 SCRAMBLED EGGS TO GO

8 SOUTHWESTERN FRITTATA WITH SPICY CORN SALSA

10 BLENDER PANCAKES WITH SWEET CINNAMON BANANAS

12 ZUCCHINI PANCAKES WITH WALNUTS AND SPICE

14 MAPLE APPLE WAFFLES

16 FRENCH TOAST WITH ORANGE MARMALADE

17 HOMEMADE GRANOLA BARS

18 LEMONY YOGURT MUFFINS

20 PEANUT BUTTER SPREAD AND JELLY ON TOAST

21 APPLE BUTTER

22 CHOCOLATE BREAKFAST SHAKE

23 ESSENTIAL SMOOTHIE

Bacon, Egg, and Cheese Sandwich

SERVES 4

A bacon, egg, and cheese sandwich is a delicious breakfast for a hearty appetite, but eating a lot of the full-fat version can be tough on the heart because of its high amounts of saturated fat. My recipe tastes hearty *and* is easy on your heart.

Nonstick cooking spray

12 slices nitrate-free turkey bacon

8 slices whole grain or whole wheat bread

4 eggs

4 egg whites

¼ cup plain, fat-free yogurt

¼ teaspoon salt

¼ teaspoon freshly ground black pepper

½ cup shredded part-skim mozzarella or reduced-fat Havarti cheese

¼ cup mild tomato salsa

Preheat the oven to 400°F. Line a large cookie sheet with aluminum foil. Coat the foil with a thin layer of cooking spray. Spread the turkey bacon out on the foil. Bake 15 to 20 minutes, until crisp. Toast the bread for 5 minutes in the oven.

In a bowl, lightly whisk the eggs, egg whites, yogurt, salt, and pepper. Heat an ovenproof medium skillet over high heat. Coat with an even layer of cooking spray and add the egg mixture. Sprinkle with the cheese and place in the oven. Bake the eggs 5 to 6 minutes, until firm.

Top half of the toast slices with salsa. Distribute the eggs on the toast. Top with the bacon and remaining toast. Serve immediately.

Skinny Secret

Everyone loves bacon, but that cured, smoked, and preserved pork is hard on the heart and the waistline. I use turkey bacon to make low-fat recipes tasty without adding tons of fat and— more importantly—without adding tons of *saturated* fat.

Per serving (1 sandwich): 453 calories, 43 g protein, 37 g carbohydrates, 15.6 g fat (4 g saturated), 294 mg cholesterol, 6 g fiber, 766 mg sodium

Bacon Sausage Omelet with Onions and Peppers

SERVES 8

I've always loved the savory taste of sausage, but I don't love all the grease that comes along with the meat. Substituting chicken sausage and adding herbs keep the omelet light and lean without sacrificing the satisfying, savory flavor.

4 egg whites

3 eggs

¼ cup plain, fat-free Greek yogurt

1 teaspoon fresh thyme leaves or chopped chives

½ teaspoon paprika

½ teaspoon salt

¼ teaspoon freshly ground black pepper

Nonstick cooking spray

1 tablespoon olive oil

2 chicken sausage links, thinly sliced

4 slices nitrate-free turkey bacon, chopped

1 green bell pepper, seeds removed, thinly sliced

1 small red or white onion, diced

1 large tomato, diced

Skinny Secret

Eggs are good for you—they're inexpensive and easy to cook. Simply substitute two egg whites for every yolk to get a filling meal that's leaner.

In a large bowl, gently whisk the egg whites, eggs, yogurt, thyme or chives, paprika, salt, and black pepper. Set aside. Heat a large skillet over high heat. Coat the skillet with cooking spray and add the olive oil. When the oil is hot but not smoking (it will shimmer), add the sausage, bacon, bell pepper, and onion. Reduce the heat to medium and cook 7 to 8 minutes, stirring occasionally, until the peppers and onions soften.

Pour the egg mixture on top and decrease the heat to low. Sprinkle on the tomato. Cover and cook on low 4 to 5 minutes, until the omelet is cooked through. Slice into eight wedges and serve immediately.

Per serving (1 wedge): 125 calories, 12 g protein, 4 g carbohydrates, 7 g fat (2 g saturated), 112 mg cholesterol, 1 g fiber, 384 mg sodium

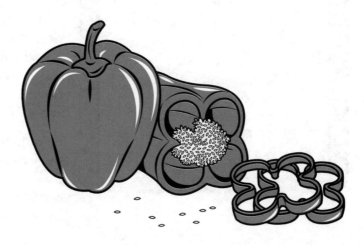

Baked Eggs and Ham

SERVES 4

Eggs have lots of nutritional value. Although I prefer to use egg whites to cut the fat in recipes, the yolks (when eaten in moderation) have plenty of good things to offer the body. If you love your eggs "dippy," or over easy, but tend to break them in a skillet, this recipe is perfect for you. Plus you're getting some veggie power!

- Nonstick cooking spray
- 2 small whole wheat pitas, peeled apart
- ½ cup pasta sauce
- 2 large tomatoes, thinly sliced
- 4 slices reduced-sodium ham
- ¼ cup packed basil leaves, torn or chopped
- 1 cup thinly sliced mushrooms
- 1 cup shredded part-skim mozzarella cheese
- ¼ cup finely chopped shallots or red onion
- 4 eggs
- ½ teaspoon salt
- ¼ teaspoon freshly ground black pepper

Skinny Secret

Fresh herbs can add impressive flavor and aroma, and they're practically calorie and fat free. Basil is my number-one choice because almost everyone loves it, and it's loaded with vitamin K that helps cuts and bruises heal.

Preheat the oven to 400°F. Coat an 8 x 12-inch baking dish with cooking spray. Arrange the pita halves in the dish. With a spatula, smear the pasta sauce over the pitas. Top with the tomato and ham. Sprinkle with the basil. Top with the mushrooms, cheese, and shallots. Make wells in the centers of the mounds and crack an egg into each. Sprinkle with salt and pepper.

Bake 15 to 18 minutes, uncovered, until the whites of the eggs are cooked through but the yolks are still soft. Lift out with a spatula onto four plates. Serve immediately.

Per serving (1 pita halve): 173 calories, 13 g protein, 17 g carbohydrates, 6 g fat (2 g saturated), 6 mg cholesterol, 2 g fiber, 701 mg sodium

Scrambled Eggs to Go

SERVES 4

I used to leave the house all the time without eating breakfast. Then around 11:00 a.m., feeling totally starved, I would pig out on anything I could grab in a hurry. Sound familiar? This is an easy, protein-packed breakfast that you can take with you and eat on the go.

 2 eggs
 3 egg whites
 ¼ cup plain, fat-free Greek yogurt
 ½ teaspoon mild chili powder
 ¼ teaspoon freshly grated nutmeg
 ¼ teaspoon freshly ground black pepper
    Nonstick cooking spray
 4 mini whole wheat pitas, toasted
 ½ cup baby spinach leaves
 4 tablespoons taco sauce

Place the eggs, egg whites, yogurt, chili powder, nutmeg, and pepper in a small bowl. Whisk until the yogurt is well incorporated into the eggs. Heat a small skillet over medium-high heat. When the skillet is hot, coat it with a layer of cooking spray. Add the eggs and cook 30 seconds, until a light brown crust starts to form. Pull the cooked edges of the eggs toward the center of the pan and cook 30 seconds more. Flip the eggs and cook an additional 30 seconds until the eggs are cooked through. Remove from the heat.

Line each pita with one-fourth of the spinach. Distribute the egg mixture among all the pitas and top with taco sauce. Serve immediately or wrap in foil and take on the road.

Per serving (1½ cups + 1 pita): 139 calories, 10 g protein, 18 g carbohydrates, 3.3 g fat (1 g saturated), 106 mg cholesterol, 2 g fiber, 338 mg sodium

Southwestern Frittata with Spicy Corn Salsa

SERVES 4

"Frittata" might sound challenging to make, but this is an easy recipe even for the novice cook. I add yogurt to keep the eggs from drying out, and as a result this omelet turns out tender and delicious. Perfect for breakfast and brunch, it can also be served as a speedy, late-night dinner. It warms up beautifully, and the beans give it a great texture and extra fiber.

SALSA

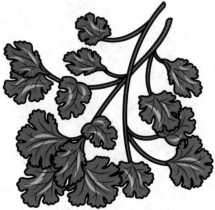

- 1 cup corn kernels, frozen (defrosted) or fresh
- ½ cup jarred tomato salsa
- 1 small jalapeño pepper, chopped
- 2 tablespoons cilantro, chopped

FRITTATA

- 1 11.5-ounce can black beans, drained and rinsed
- 4 egg whites
- 2 eggs
- ½ cup plain, fat-free Greek yogurt
- ¼ cup packed cilantro leaves
- ¼ teaspoon freshly ground black pepper
     Nonstick cooking spray
- 2 teaspoons olive oil
- 2 jalapeño peppers, seeds removed, chopped
- 3 scallions, thinly sliced
- ¼ teaspoon salt
- 1 cup baby spinach leaves, packed
- ¼ cup shredded part-skim mozzarella cheese
- 4 tablespoons fat-free sour cream

Preheat the oven to 350°F. In a small bowl, mix the corn, salsa, jalapeño, and cilantro. Set aside.

In a large bowl, stir the beans, egg whites, eggs, yogurt, cilantro, and black pepper until well combined. Set aside. Heat a large skillet over high heat. Coat with cooking spray and add the olive oil. When the oil is hot but not smoking (it will shimmer), add the jalapeños, scallions, and salt. Reduce the heat to medium and cook 5 to 6 minutes, stirring occasionally, until the peppers and onions soften. Add the spinach and cook an additional minute, until the spinach begins to wilt.

Pour the egg mixture on top and decrease the heat to low. Sprinkle the eggs with cheese, cover, and cook on low 4 to 5 minutes, until the egg mixture is cooked through. Slice into four wedges and transfer to four plates. Top each frittata with a spoonful of the salsa and the sour cream. Serve immediately.

Per serving (1 wedge): 240 calories, 19 g protein, 29 g carbohydrates, 7 g fat (1.2 g saturated), 107 mg cholesterol, 7 g fiber, 774 mg sodium

Skinny Secret

Sharing a healthy brunch is a great way to spend quality time with friends and family—and even beginning cooks get this frittata right every time.

Blender Pancakes with Sweet Cinnamon Bananas

MAKES 8 PANCAKES

Want to get your kids to eat more whole grains without a fight? Serve these delicious whole wheat pancakes. They are appealingly thin and have a wonderful texture. Lose the banana and tuck in a slice of turkey to invent a new lunch-box favorite. These pancakes can be cooked in advance and gently reheated in a 200°F oven.

- 1 cup low-fat (1 percent) buttermilk
- ½ cup whole wheat flour
- 1 egg
- ½ teaspoon canola oil
- ¼ teaspoon ground nutmeg
- ¼ teaspoon ground cardamom
- ¼ teaspoon salt
- Nonstick cooking spray
- 4 medium bananas (about 1½ pounds)
- 1 teaspoon ground cinnamon

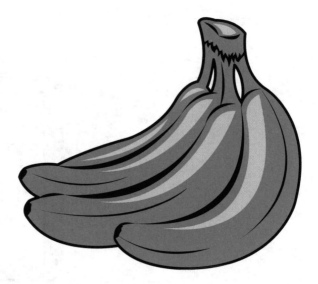

Place the buttermilk, flour, egg, oil, nutmeg, cardamom, and salt in a blender. Blend on high until smooth, about 1 minute. Cover and refrigerate the batter at least 1 hour or overnight.

Heat a large griddle over high heat. Coat with an even layer of cooking spray. Spoon out 3-tablespoon rounds of batter onto the griddle, leaving about 1 inch between each pancake. Cook 2 to 3 minutes, until tiny bubbles start to form on the surface and the edges become crisp. Flip and cook an additional minute or two, until each pancake is cooked through. Transfer the pancakes to a plate and repeat with remaining batter.

Cut the bananas in half lengthwise. Coat them with cooking spray and sprinkle with cinnamon. Place them on the griddle. Cook 3 to 4 minutes, turning once, until the bananas are soft and lightly charred. Slice them and serve immediately with the pancakes.

Per serving (1 pancake): 105 calories, 4 g protein, 21 g carbohydrates, 1.6 g fat (0.5 g saturated), 28 mg cholesterol, 3 g fiber, 44 mg sodium

Skinny Secret

One of the easiest ways to start your family on whole grains is to add the good grains to pancake batter, because the swap doesn't change the texture of the pancakes much.

Zucchini Pancakes with Walnuts and Spice

SERVES 4

The more you cook, the more you'll find that some vegetables work as well in sweet recipes as they do in savory. Zucchini and carrots are two good examples. These pancakes are sweet and spicy, and they're a perfect way to use an overabundance of the summer squash.

$\frac{2}{3}$ cup all-purpose flour

$\frac{1}{4}$ cup whole wheat flour

  2 tablespoons chopped walnuts

  2 tablespoons ground flaxseed

  1 teaspoon baking powder

$\frac{1}{4}$ teaspoon baking soda

$\frac{1}{2}$ teaspoon ground cinnamon

$\frac{1}{8}$ teaspoon ground cloves

$\frac{1}{8}$ teaspoon ground nutmeg

$\frac{1}{8}$ teaspoon salt

  2 large eggs

  1 cup low-fat (1 percent) buttermilk

$\frac{1}{2}$ small zucchini, grated (about $\frac{1}{2}$ cup)

  1 small banana, mashed (about $\frac{1}{3}$ cup)

  1 small carrot, grated (about $\frac{1}{2}$ cup)

  2 tablespoons honey

$\frac{1}{4}$ cup water

     Nonstick cooking spray

Combine the flours, walnuts, flaxseed, baking powder, baking soda, cinnamon, cloves, nutmeg, and salt in a large mixing bowl. Stir well to combine. Make a well in the center and add the eggs, buttermilk, zucchini, banana, carrot, honey, and water. Stir the wet ingredients in the well, gently incorporating the flour as you stir, until a loose batter begins to form. Continue to stir about 20 turns, until most of the flour is incorporated. Do not overstir; there will be some dry spots.

Coat a large skillet or griddle with cooking spray. Place the skillet or griddle over medium-high heat. Using a 1/4-cup measure, pour out the batter, leaving about 1 inch between pancakes. Cook 3 to 4 minutes, until the tops of the pancakes begin to form tiny bubbles. Flip the pancakes and cook another 2 to 3 minutes, until the pancakes are cooked through. Transfer to a plate and repeat with the remaining batter.

To keep the pancakes warm, cover the plate with aluminum foil and place it in a 200°F oven for up to 1 hour. To freeze, cool the pancakes completely on a wire rack, then seal them in a zipper-lock bag and store in the freezer for up to 6 months.

Per serving (2 pancakes): 241 calories, 10 g protein, 34 g carbohydrates, 7.7 g fat (1.6 g saturated), 110 mg cholesterol, 4 g fiber, 366 mg sodium

Skinny Secret

Adding grated vegetables to most main dishes—rather than serving veggies as sides—encourages children to accept vegetables as an integral component of the meal.

Maple Apple Waffles

SERVES 8

With all the confusion about which products on the market actually contain whole grains, the easiest way to make sure that you're getting real grains is to make your food yourself. These tasty waffles freeze well, and you can pop them in a toaster oven or preheated oven for a fast breakfast. I like to save the leftovers and make an afternoon sandwich for my husband with turkey breast and a slice of Swiss cheese.

    1 large apple, such as Golden Delicious or Gala, cored and cubed
    2 tablespoons balsamic vinegar
    2 tablespoons maple syrup
    1 teaspoon vanilla extract
    4 egg whites
    2 cups fat-free milk
    2 tablespoons trans-fat-free margarine, melted
    2 cups soft whole wheat flour, such as white whole wheat
      or whole wheat pastry
    2 tablespoons ground flaxseed
    2 teaspoons baking powder
    1 teaspoon ground cinnamon
  ¼ teaspoon salt
    Nonstick cooking spray

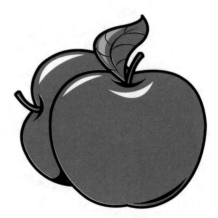

Preheat a waffle iron on high. Meanwhile, place the apples, vinegar, maple syrup, and vanilla in a large bowl. Stir until the apples turn slightly brown from the vinegar. Add the egg whites, milk, and margarine.

Place the flour, flaxseed, baking powder, cinnamon, and salt in a fine-mesh sieve. Shake the flour mixture over the wet ingredients. Using a spatula, stir the flour until a soft batter begins to form, about 10 turns.

Coat the waffle iron with cooking spray. Pour 1 cup of batter in the center of the iron and close the lid. Cook until the waffle is golden and crisp (the lid should release easily), 5 to 6 minutes. Repeat with the remaining batter. Serve immediately.

Per serving (1 waffle): 189 calories, 8 g protein, 33 g carbohydrates, 3.2 g fat (0.8 g saturated), 1 mg cholesterol, 4 g fiber, 251 mg sodium

Skinny Secret

A lot of people skip breakfast because they are rushed or just not hungry. This can make you overeat at lunch and create crazy cravings throughout the day.

French Toast with Orange Marmalade

SERVES 4

Whole grains can lower the risk of diabetes and heart disease and help you maintain your weight because they make you feel full longer. Without sacrificing flavor, I've swapped whole wheat bread for white bread in this French toast. French toast is great with a hint of sweetness, but you don't need to overload it with a ton of sugar. Marmalade and orange zest lend plenty of flavor.

  1 cup fat-free milk
  2 eggs
  2 egg whites
  ¼ cup orange marmalade
  1 teaspoon ground cardamom
  2 large oranges (about ¾ pound)
     Nonstick cooking spray
  8 slices whole wheat or whole grain sandwich bread

In a large bowl, whisk the milk, eggs, egg whites, orange marmalade, and cardamom. Using a zester or microplane, zest the orange directly into the bowl with the eggs. Whisk the mixture until smooth. Slice off the remaining orange peel. Working over a bowl, use a small paring knife to free the orange sections from their membrane. Discard the membranes. Set the orange sections aside.

Heat two large skillets over medium-high heat. Coat both with cooking spray. Dip each bread slice into the egg mixture; transfer four slices to each skillet. Cook 3 to 4 minutes, until the bread begins to brown. Coat the tops of all the slices with a thick layer of cooking spray and flip. Cook 4 to 5 minutes more, until the bread is no longer wet in the center. Serve immediately with the orange sections.

Skinny Secret

A zester or microplane has tiny holes that create thin strips from foods. This handy tool eliminates the need for and danger from using a small knife.

Per serving (2 slices): 298 calories, 15 g protein, 51 g carbohydrates, 4.5 g fat (1.2 g saturated), 107 mg cholesterol, 6 g fiber, 371 mg sodium

Homemade Granola Bars

MAKES 8 BARS

When I was a teenager trying to catch the eye of a neighborhood boy I had a crush on, I worked so hard to lose weight and get fit. Back then I didn't know that so-called healthy granola bars and cereal could be calorie bombs, and I was confused when the pounds never melted away. Oftentimes, processed snack bars contain loads of sugar as well as additives like trans-fats that can be detrimental to your health. Here's a bar without all the bad stuff!

Nonstick cooking spray

2 tablespoons reduced-fat peanut butter

3 egg whites

1 tablespoon unsulfured molasses

1½ cups rolled oats

¼ cup prunes, chopped

2 tablespoons ground flaxseed

2 tablespoons pumpkin seeds

1 tablespoon sesame seeds

1 teaspoon pumpkin pie spice

Preheat the oven to 350°F. Line an 8 x 8-inch baking dish with aluminum foil. Coat the foil with cooking spray. Place the peanut butter, egg whites, and molasses in a large bowl. Mash the peanut butter into the eggs and molasses with the back of a wooden spoon until a smooth mixture forms.

Add the oats, prunes, flaxseed, pumpkin seeds, sesame seeds, and pumpkin pie spice. Mix well and transfer to the baking dish. Press into an even layer with a rubber spatula. Coat the top of the batter with a light coating of cooking spray. Bake 40 to 45 minutes, until the oats are golden and firm. Cool completely before cutting into eight bars.

Per serving (1 bar): 131 calories, 6 g protein, 17 g carbohydrates, 4 g fat (0.4 g saturated), 0 mg cholesterol, 3 g fiber, 25 mg sodium

Lemony Yogurt Muffins

MAKES 12 MUFFINS

Store-bought muffins can be fat traps, delivering a whopping one-third of your fat intake for the day. If you love to have fresh muffins in the morning, make this batter in advance and freeze it in individual paper cupcake liners, then just pop one into the oven when you head into the shower. It will be wonderfully warm by the time you're ready to go.

  1 cup white whole wheat flour
  1 cup all-purpose flour
  ½ teaspoon baking powder
  1 teaspoon baking soda
  ¼ teaspoon salt
  ½ cup granulated sugar
  ⅓ cup reduced-fat, trans-fat–free margarine
  2 egg whites
  1 cup plain, fat-free Greek yogurt
  2 lemons, zested and juiced

ADD-INS (CHOOSE JUST ONE TO KEEP CALORIES IN CHECK)

  Crunchy: ¼ cup chopped almonds or walnuts
  Fruity: ¼ cup chopped cranberries, ¼ chopped prunes
  High fiber: 2 tablespoons wheat germ

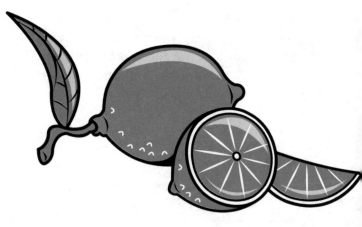

Grease and flour a 12-cup muffin tin or line the cups of a muffin tin with paper liners. Combine the flours, baking powder, baking soda, and salt in a large bowl or zipper-lock bag. Stir or shake well to combine.

In a medium bowl, mash the sugar and margarine with the back of a wooden spoon until smooth. Stir in the egg whites, yogurt, lemon zest, lemon juice, and one of the add-ins, if using. Add the flour mixture and stir with a wooden spoon until a batter forms, about 10 strokes. Don't overmix, otherwise your muffins will be tough.

Fill the muffin cups three-fourths full. Cover with a tight layer of aluminum foil and freeze for up to 1 month. Bake at 350°F for 20 to 25 minutes, adding a minute or two if the batter is frozen, until the muffins spring back to the touch. Cool completely before storing in an airtight container for up to 3 days.

Per serving (1 muffin, plain): 157 calories, 5 g protein, 25 g carbohydrates, 4 g fat (1.2 g saturated), 0 mg cholesterol, 1 g fiber, 227 mg sodium

With nuts: 172 calories, 5 g protein, 26 g carbohydrates, 5.9 g fat (1.4 g saturated), 0 mg cholesterol, 1 g fiber, 227 mg sodium

With fruit: 167 calories, 5 g protein, 28 g carbohydrates, 4.3 g fat (1.2 g saturated), 0 mg cholesterol, 1.5 g fiber, 227 mg sodium

With wheat germ: 161 calories, 5 g protein, 26 g carbohydrates, 4.3 g fat (1.2 g saturated), 0 mg cholesterol, 1 g fiber, 227 mg sodium

Peanut Butter Spread and Jelly on Toast

SERVES 4

Everyone loves the sweet-and-salty combo of peanut butter and jelly. I figured out a way to add more nutrition to this classic while cutting back on fat. This "jam" is made without the zero-nutrition high fructose corn syrup commonly found in commercial products; plus I added whole grains, omega-3 fatty acids from the flaxseed, and freshly cooked fruit.

- ½ pint fresh blueberries
- 1 tablespoon granulated sugar
- ¼ cup reduced-fat creamy peanut butter
- ¼ cup plain, fat-free Greek yogurt
- 1 tablespoon ground flaxseed
- 4 slices whole wheat or whole grain bread

Place the berries and sugar in a small saucepan. Cook over high heat until the berries begin to pop and a thick sauce starts to form. Add 1 or 2 tablespoons of water if the mixture starts to stick to the pan.

Meanwhile, stir the peanut butter, yogurt, and flaxseed together in a small bowl. Toast the bread, top with the peanut butter mixture, and dot with the blueberry "jam."

Skinny Secret

Blueberries have a natural sweetness and are high in beneficial antioxidants, which can lead to beautiful skin and a healthy heart. They also make a wonderful substitute for calorie-laden sugar bombs at breakfast, snack time, and dessert.

Per serving (1 slice): 216 calories, 9 g protein, 29 g carbohydrates, 8 g fat (1.5 g saturated), 0 mg cholesterol, 4 g fiber, 263 mg sodium

Apple Butter

MAKES 1 CUP BUTTER

Thick, rich-tasting apple butter can take the place of a pat of (high in saturated fat) butter on your morning toast. You can even add a dollop to a scoop of frozen yogurt for added flavor without fat.

3 apples (about 1¼ pounds), peeled, cored, and sliced
½ cup apple cider
½ cup firmly packed light brown sugar
2 strips of orange zest, each 2½ inches long
2 teaspoons ground cinnamon
½ teaspoon ground allspice
¼ teaspoon ground cloves
1 star anise pod
¼ teaspoon salt

In a large saucepan, cook the apples in the cider over moderate heat, stirring occasionally, for 30 minutes or until tender. Carefully transfer the apples and their liquid to a food processor and process until smooth. Transfer the mixture along with the sugar, orange zest, cinnamon, allspice, cloves, star anise pod, and salt to a slow cooker or rice cooker.

Cook the mixture over very low heat, stirring occasionally, for about 2 hours or until very thick. If you are using the rice cooker, add 1 to 2 tablespoons of water if the mixture begins to stick. Remove the star anise. Cool completely before transferring the apple butter to an airtight container. Refrigerate for up to 2 weeks.

Per serving (1 tablespoon): 45 calories, 0 g protein,
12 g carbohydrates, 0 g fat, 0 mg cholesterol,
1 g fiber, 38 mg sodium

Chocolate Breakfast Shake

SERVES 4

When I was a teen, I was hooked on creamy, smooth chocolate milk. I used to drink it to wash down a bag of chips at least 3 or 4 times a week. This lower-fat version of a chocolate shake tastes just as rich, and it has a lot more to offer than just the calcium from milk—including cultures from yogurt and potassium from banana.

    1   cup plain, fat-free Greek yogurt
    1½ cups fat-free milk
    1   medium banana (about 7 ounces)
    2   cups ice
    2   tablespoons unsweetened cocoa powder
    2   tablespoons honey or granulated sugar

Combine all the ingredients in a blender. Cover and blend until smooth, about 1 minute. Distribute the shake among four glasses and serve immediately.

Per serving (1¼ cups): 126 calories, 9 g protein, 24 g carbohydrates, 0.6 g fat (0.3 g saturated), 0 mg cholesterol, 2 g fiber, 62 mg sodium

Skinny Secret

Store-bought diet shakes are often expensive, and they can sit on the shelves for years. Make your shakes with fresh, seasonal, locally grown ingredients instead. You'll save money and you'll save on calories!

Essential Smoothie

SERVES 2

Don't rely on an artificial, preservative-laden protein bar or diet shake as a snack or quick breakfast. Instead, try a smoothie. It's a cinch to prepare, and this one is packed with essential vitamins your body can easily absorb. Your skin and hair will thank you.

> 1 cup plain, fat-free Greek yogurt
> ½ cup carrot juice
> ½ cup orange juice
> 1 small banana
> 2 tablespoons ground flaxseed
> 2 tablespoons pumpkin seeds
> 8 ice cubes (about 1 cup)

Place the yogurt, carrot juice, orange juice, banana, flaxseed, pumpkin seeds, and ice cubes in a blender. Blend on high until smooth and serve immediately.

Per serving (1¼ cups): 268 calories, 17 g protein, 30 g carbohydrates, 9.7 g fat (1.5 g saturated), 0 mg cholesterol, 4 g fiber, 87 mg sodium

Skinny Secret

Flaxseed can be one of your secret weapons because it has a mild flavor, looks like ground sesame, and is a great source of healthful omega-3 fatty acids, soluble fiber, and protein. Store flaxseed in the fridge so the essential oils in the ground seeds don't spoil. Preferably cook with ground flaxseed, since the whole seeds tend to pass through your system without being digested.

Soups,
Appetizers, and
Snacks

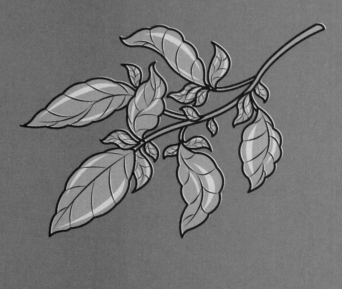

27 BUTTERNUT SQUASH SOUP WITH COCONUT MILK

28 FRENCH ONION SOUP WITH CHEESY WHOLE WHEAT CROUTONS

30 GARLICKY BLACK BEAN SOUP

32 FOUR FOOD GROUPS MINESTRONE

34 ALARMINGLY GOOD LOW-FAT CHILI

36 "CREAM" OF BROCCOLI SOUP WITH CHEDDAR

37 SHRIMP AND CORN CHOWDER

38 TEN-MINUTE CHICKEN NOODLE SOUP

39 POOLSIDE SOUP

40 BACON-WRAPPED DATES

41 CREAMY MEXICAN BEAN DIP WITH WHOLE GRAIN TORTILLA CHIPS

42 NACHOS GRANDE WITH PICKLED JALAPEÑO SALSA

44 HOT "WINGS" WITH SPICY SAUCE

45 PARTY DIP SERVED WITH WHOLE WHEAT PITA

46 PARTY MIX WITH SPICED NUTS AND WHOLE GRAIN CEREAL

Butternut Squash Soup with Coconut Milk

SERVES 8

Pureed soups are perfect ways to satisfy your craving for something rich. My friend Chef Geraldo from Dino and Harry's Steakhouse Restaurant makes his pumpkin soup creamy and rich tasting with coconut milk, but I use the light coconut milk version.

- 2 teaspoons olive oil
- 1 red onion, chopped
- 2 garlic cloves, minced
- 1 15-ounce can reduced-sodium, fat-free chicken broth
- 1 3-pound butternut squash, cubed and diced
- ¼ teaspoon freshly grated nutmeg
- ¼ teaspoon mild chili powder
- ¼ teaspoon salt
- 1 15-ounce can light coconut milk
- ¼ cup unsweetened shredded coconut
- ¼ cup toasted chopped pistachios or peanuts

Heat the oil in a large stockpot over medium-high heat. Add the onions and garlic, and cook 8 to 10 minutes, stirring often, adding 2 to 3 table-spoons of the chicken broth so the onions do not stick. Add the butternut squash, nutmeg, chili powder, and salt, and cook an additional 2 to 3 minutes, until the spices become fragrant.

Add the coconut milk and remaining broth. Bring to a slow simmer, stirring once or twice. Cook 10 to 15 minutes, until the soup reduces slightly. Using an immersion blender, puree the soup in the pot until smooth, or transfer in batches to a blender to puree. Sprinkle the soup with the coconut and nuts and serve immediately.

Skinny Secret

You gotta love homemade soups. They are the perfect vehicle for healthy meals, filling yet packed with veggies, and an easy sell for kids. There's no need to dump heavy cream into them—a little mashed white or sweet potato can make them just as creamy!

Per serving (1¼ cups): 171 calories, 4 g protein, 22 g carbohydrates, 9 g fat (5 g saturated), 0 mg cholesterol, 4 g fiber, 207 mg sodium

French Onion Soup with Cheesy Whole Wheat Croutons

SERVES 8

French Onion Soup is a staple in French-style bistros, but eating this dish in restaurants all the time can really pack on the pounds, since most eateries enrich the soup with lots of high-calorie items like butter and oils. Caramelized onions are easy to make and have a naturally sweet and creamy texture. If you have a food processor, you can easily slice the onions with a slicer attachment to make the prep even simpler.

1 tablespoon olive oil

4 large mild onions (about 3 pounds), such as Vidalia, thinly sliced

1 tablespoon dark brown sugar

2 32-ounce cartons or cans reduced-sodium beef broth

8 slices (about 8 ounces) whole wheat baguette or other crusty whole wheat bread, cut into 1-inch cubes

Nonstick cooking spray

2 tablespoons grated Parmesan cheese

½ teaspoon garlic powder

½ teaspoon onion powder

¼ teaspoon paprika

¼ teaspoon freshly ground black pepper

1 cup shredded part-skim mozzarella cheese

Heat a large stockpot over high heat. Add the oil and the onions. Cook 5 to 6 minutes, until the onions start to soften and brown slightly. Add the brown sugar and lower the heat to medium low. Continue to cook 20 to 25 minutes, until the onions are very soft and brown, adding tablespoons of the beef broth if the onions start to stick to the pan. Add the remaining beef broth and bring the mixture to a slow simmer, cooking 10 minutes longer.

Meanwhile, place the bread on a sheet of waxed paper. Coat the bread with a layer of cooking spray and sprinkle on the Parmesan, garlic powder, onion powder, paprika, and pepper. Coat a large skillet with cooking spray and place over medium

French Onion Soup with Cheesy
Whole Wheat Croutons, page 28

Mac and Cheese with Shredded Chicken
and Cauliflower, page 52

heat. Add the bread cubes and top them with another layer of cooking spray. Cook 2 to 3 minutes, turning occasionally with a spatula, until the bread cubes are nicely browned.

Preheat oven to 400°F. Place eight heatproof bowls or coffee mugs on a baking tray. Divide the soup among the cups. Sprinkle with the mozzarella and bake 5 to 10 minutes, until the cheese is melted. Remove the tray from the oven and sprinkle the soup with the croutons. Serve immediately.

Per serving (1 cup soup + cheese garnish + ¼ cup croutons): 211 calories, 10 g protein, 31 g carbohydrates, 5 g fat (2.1 g saturated), 10 mg cholesterol, 4 g fiber, 290 mg sodium

Skinny Secret

Three tips to tweak bad eating habits: Drink an extra glass of water, eat out one fewer meal every week, and swap your afternoon candy with something healthier.

Garlicky Black Bean Soup

SERVES 8

My father loves my Garlicky Black Bean Soup, but he prefers a looser texture to the smoothly blended version. So I simply mash some of the beans with a wooden spoon before I serve the soup to him. The cocoa powder in this recipe might seem strange, but it creates a richer color. I added eggs to increase the protein content, making this dish a complete meal for vegetarians who eat eggs.

1 tablespoon olive oil

1 small red onion (about 1 cup), chopped

4 garlic cloves, minced

2 tablespoons mild chili powder

1 tablespoon unsweetened cocoa powder

1 tablespoon ground cumin

1 small dried red chile or 1 teaspoon red chile flakes

2 sprigs fresh thyme

2 15-ounce cans low-sodium black beans, well drained and rinsed

2 quarts low-sodium, fat-free chicken or vegetable broth

8 whole wheat or whole grain flour tortillas

2 limes, juiced

8 eggs

8 tablespoons jarred tomato salsa

4 scallions, thinly sliced

¼ cup cilantro leaves, chopped

In a large stockpot, heat the oil over medium-high heat until hot but not smoking. Add the onions and garlic and cook 5 to 6 minutes, stirring occasionally, until the onions soften but do not brown. Add the chili powder, cocoa, cumin, dried chile or chile flakes, and thyme. Continue to cook 1 to 2 minutes, stirring often, until the spices release their aroma.

Increase the heat to high and add the drained beans and the chicken or vegetable broth. Cover the pot and bring the soup to a slow boil. Reduce the heat to a simmer and continue cooking 15 or 20 minutes, until the beans are tender and have started to break apart.

Meanwhile, wrap the tortillas in aluminum foil and place them in a 400°F oven or toaster oven for 5 to 10 minutes to warm.

Add the lime juice to the soup and stir well. Carefully crack the eggs into the soup. Cover and reduce to a slow simmer. Allow the eggs to cook 7 to 8 minutes, until the yolks are still soft but the whites are firm. Using a large ladle, lift out about a cup of the soup with one egg per bowl. Top with salsa, scallions, and cilantro. Serve immediately with the warmed tortillas.

Per serving (1¼ cup soup + 1 tortilla): 314 calories, 17 g protein, 39 g carbohydrates, 10 g fat (2 g saturated), 212 mg cholesterol, 8 g fiber, 548 mg sodium

Skinny Secret

Maintaining weight is easier when you think a little more about portion sizes. One small change, like using a smaller bowl, sustained over months, will make a huge difference!

Four Food Groups Minestrone

SERVES 6

Soup can make a healthy meal when it features plenty of veggies and is low in sodium. I call this Four Food Groups Minestrone because it has almost everything in one meal: veggies, meat, dairy, and grains. It even includes a little wine that adds much flavor—a good way to use up the last of a wine bottle.

1	tablespoon olive oil
1	red onion, chopped
2	carrots, peeled and chopped
2	celery stalks, chopped
2	garlic cloves, chopped
$\frac{1}{2}$	teaspoon red pepper flakes
1	cup dry red or white wine
1	large tomato, seeded and chopped
48	ounces reduced-sodium, fat-free chicken stock
2	cups water
1	bay leaf
1	cup whole grain pasta, such as rotini, penne, or shells
$\frac{1}{2}$	pound ground sirloin
$\frac{1}{4}$	cup grated Parmesan cheese
$\frac{1}{4}$	cup fat-free milk
1	egg white
$\frac{1}{2}$	cup whole wheat bread crumbs (1 slice whole wheat bread)
2	cups chopped collard greens
1	15-ounce can cannellini beans, red kidney beans, or chickpeas, well drained and rinsed
$\frac{1}{4}$	cup chopped fresh basil

In a large stockpot, warm the olive oil over medium-high heat. Add the onions, carrots, celery, garlic, and pepper flakes. Cook, stirring occasionally, until softened, 7 to 8 minutes. Add the wine and tomato and bring to a boil. Stir in the stock, water, bay leaf, and pasta. Cook 10 to 15 minutes, until the pasta is nearly cooked.

In a medium bowl, mix the sirloin, Parmesan, milk, egg white, and bread crumbs until well combined. Roll the meat mixture into ½-inch meatballs and place them on a sheet of waxed paper. Increase the stockpot heat to high. Carefully drop the meatballs into the soup, stirring gently. Add the collards and beans. Cover and simmer 10 minutes, until the meatballs are cooked through. Discard the bay leaf. Add the basil before serving.

Per serving (1½ cups): 254 calories, 17 g protein, 26 g carbohydrates, 6 g fat (2 g saturated), 27 mg cholesterol, 5 g fiber, 359 mg sodium

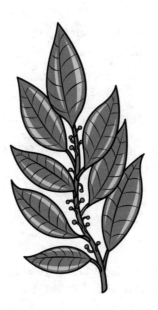

Alarmingly Good Low-Fat Chili

SERVES 4

I'm a meat lover. I grew up eating lots of beef, and the savory taste of steak is one of my favorite flavors. But eating lots of beef can be a fattening way to get your protein fix. This recipe is a great way to feed a crowd or host a party for hearty eaters who love meat; no need to tell them it's made with turkey instead of beef!

- 1 tablespoon olive oil
- 1 green bell pepper, chopped
- 1 red bell pepper, chopped
- 1 small red or white onion, chopped
- 4 garlic cloves, minced
- 1 pound ground turkey breast
- ¼ teaspoon salt
- ½ teaspoon freshly ground black pepper
- 2 tablespoons mild chili powder
- 2 tablespoons cumin powder
- 1 canned chipotle chile in adobo sauce
- 1 tablespoon adobo sauce
- 1 28-ounce can crushed organic tomatoes
- 1 15-ounce can reduced-sodium, fat-free chicken broth
- 1 16-ounce can red kidney beans, drained and rinsed
- 2 tablespoons ground flaxseed

CHIPOTLE CREAM TOPPING (OPTIONAL)

- ½ cup reduced-fat sour cream
- 1 garlic clove
- 1 lime, zested and juiced

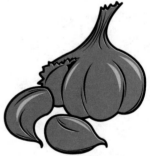

Heat the oil olive in a large stockpot over medium-high heat. Add the bell peppers, onions, and garlic. Cook 6 to 7 minutes, until the onions start to soften. Sprinkle the ground turkey with salt and black pepper. Increase the heat to high and add the turkey to the stockpot. Cook 5 to 6 minutes, stirring occasionally, until the turkey browns. Add the chili powder, cumin, chipotle, and adobo sauce and cook 1 to 2 minutes more, stirring once or twice, until the spices become fragrant.

Add the tomatoes and chicken broth. Bring to a slow boil, breaking up the tomatoes with a spoon. Cover and reduce to a simmer; cook 15 to 20 minutes, until the turkey is cooked through and the liquid is slightly reduced.

Meanwhile, make the Chipotle Cream Topping, if using. Stir the sour cream, garlic, lime zest, and lime juice in a small bowl. Cover and refrigerate.

Stir the beans and flaxseed into the chili and cook uncovered 5 additional minutes, until the beans are warm. Serve immediately with the chipotle cream, if desired.

Per serving (2 cups): 350 calories, 39 g protein, 36 g carbohydrates, 8.4 g fat (0.8 g saturated), 45 mg cholesterol, 12 g fiber, 738 mg sodium

Note: Adobo is the Spanish word for seasoning or marinade. It's a luscious, low-fat spicy sauce that adds heat and the healing power of hot chiles. Find it in the international section of the supermarket.

Skinny Secret

Having a hard time getting your family to eat vegetables? Chilis and soups are great ways to pack in the veggies without the complaints.

"Cream" of Broccoli Soup with Cheddar

SERVES 8

My father used to own a deli where he made the most delectable cream of broccoli soup loaded with cheese and heavy cream! Here is my skinny version, with reduced levels of saturated fat. You can serve this soup as part of a healthy lunch or dinner.

1 tablespoon olive oil

2 small red potatoes, peeled and cubed

1 small onion, chopped

2 garlic cloves, chopped

1 head broccoli, stalk chopped and florets set aside

½ teaspoon salt

1 32-ounce carton or can reduced-sodium, fat-free chicken broth

2 teaspoons curry powder

¼ teaspoon freshly ground black pepper

1 6-ounce package baby spinach

¼ cup reduced-fat sour cream or reduced-fat yogurt

1 cup shredded reduced-fat (2 percent) Cheddar cheese

Heat the olive oil in a large stockpot. Add the potatoes, onions, garlic, broccoli stalk, and salt. Cook 5 to 6 minutes, until the vegetables start to soften. Add 1 to 2 tablespoons of the broth if the onions start to stick or brown too quickly. Add the broth, curry powder, and pepper and bring to a slow boil.

Reduce to a simmer and cover. Cook 15 to 20 minutes, until the potatoes and broccoli stalks are tender. Add the spinach and sour cream or yogurt. Using an immersion blender, puree the soup in the stockpot until smooth, or transfer it in batches to a countertop blender to puree. Add the broccoli florets and cook an additional 1 to 2 minutes, until they are tender. Ladle the soup into eight serving bowls and sprinkle each with 2 tablespoons of the Cheddar cheese. Serve immediately.

Per serving (1 cup): 126 calories, 9 g protein, 11 g carbohydrates, 6.6 g fat (2.8 g saturated), 13 mg cholesterol, 3 g fiber, 350 mg sodium

Shrimp and Corn Chowder

SERVES 8

Shrimp and corn go naturally together, since they both have a sweet, mild flavor. I call for frozen shrimp because it can be less expensive and is easier to prepare if you are not used to cooking seafood.

1	tablespoon olive oil
3	slices nitrate-free turkey bacon, chopped
1	yellow onion, chopped
2	celery stalks, chopped
2	carrots, chopped
$\frac{1}{2}$	teaspoon garlic powder
$\frac{1}{4}$	teaspoon cayenne pepper
$\frac{1}{4}$	teaspoon freshly ground black pepper
2	russet potatoes, peeled and cut into 1-inch cubes
1	32-ounce carton or can reduced-sodium, fat-free chicken broth
3	ears of corn, kernels removed, or 2 cups frozen corn, defrosted
$\frac{1}{4}$	cup half-and-half
1	pound frozen shrimp, defrosted and peeled

Heat the olive oil in a large stockpot over medium-high heat. Add the bacon, onions, celery, carrots, garlic powder, cayenne, and black pepper. Cook 5 to 6 minutes, until the onions and celery begin to soften. Add the potatoes and chicken broth. Bring to a slow boil. Reduce the heat to a simmer and cover.

Cook 15 to 20 minutes, until the potatoes are tender. Mash the potatoes slightly with the back of a spoon. Add the corn kernels, half-and-half, and shrimp. Simmer an additional 5 minutes, until the corn is tender and the shrimp is cooked through. Serve immediately.

Per serving (1$\frac{1}{2}$ cups): 145 calories, 8 g protein, 23 g carbohydrates, 3.6 g fat (1 g saturated), 18 mg cholesterol, 3 g fiber, 294 mg sodium

Ten-Minute Chicken Noodle Soup

SERVE 8

When I worked as a private chef for families, I would often have to whip up a quick chicken noodle soup to soothe an unexpected cold—especially in the fall and winter months. Soups can be so healthful because they are packed with veggies, and a warm broth can help you feel full with fewer calories.

2	tablespoons olive oil
3	carrots, peeled and thinly sliced
2	celery stalks, thinly sliced
1	small red onion, chopped
1	teaspoon lemon zest (from 1 medium lemon)
1	teaspoon mild chili powder
½	teaspoon ground celery seed
½	teaspoon ground coriander
¼	teaspoon freshly ground black pepper
1	32-ounce carton or can reduced-sodium, fat-free chicken broth
1	cup water
1	cup small egg noodles
1	rotisserie chicken (about 3 pounds), skin discarded and meat shredded
¼	cup packed fresh tarragon leaves

Heat the oil in a large stockpot over medium-high heat. Add the carrots, celery, and onions. Cook 4 to 5 minutes, until the vegetables start to soften. Add the lemon zest, chili powder, celery seed, coriander, and pepper. Cook 1 additional minute, until the veggies are cooked through and the carrots are soft.

Add the chicken broth, water, and noodles to the vegetables. Bring the broth mixture to a boil and cook 3 to 4 additional minutes, until the noodles are tender. Add the chicken and tarragon. Stir to combine and serve immediately.

Per serving (1¼ cups): 203 calories, 23 g protein, 9 g carbohydrates, 9 g fat (2 g saturated), 69 mg cholesterol, 1 g fiber, 372 mg sodium

Shrimp and Corn Chowder, page 37

Breaded Zucchini with Marinara
Dipping Sauce, page 108

Poolside Soup

SERVES 8

I named this Poolside Soup because it's light and packed with velvety, cool flavors that can refresh you on a hot day. It's the perfect fast lunch—and one that won't give you the belly bulge we all want to avoid during swimsuit weather.

4 cups green grapes

2 ripe Hass avocados, peeled

2 kiwifruits, peeled and quartered

2 medium shallots or ½ medium red onion, quartered

¼ cup red wine vinegar

1 cup fresh mint leaves

½ cup slivered almonds

1 teaspoon salt

¼ cup cold water

Place the grapes, avocados, kiwis, shallots or red onions, vinegar, mint, almonds, and salt in a food processor. Add the water and pulse the mixture until smooth. Serve at room temperature or chill covered in an airtight container for at least 1 hour or up to 2 days.

Per serving (1 cup): 137 calories, 3 g protein, 15 g carbohydrates, 9 g fat (1 g saturated), 0 mg cholesterol, 4 g fiber, 296 mg sodium

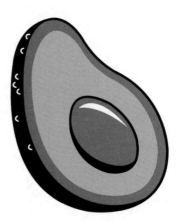

Bacon-Wrapped Dates

SERVES 4

I ate these dates while traveling in Spain, but the Spanish version is wrapped in greasy bacon that never seems to crisp up. This version has all the flavors with almost no saturated fat.

Nonstick cooking spray

8 whole toasted almonds

4 dried dates, such as Medjool, pits removed, torn in half lengthwise

8 slices nitrate-free turkey bacon

8 teaspoons fat-free sour cream

8 endive leaves

Preheat the oven to 400°F. Coat a large baking sheet with cooking spray. Press an almond into each date half. Wrap a slice of bacon around each date half and place the wrapped dates on the baking sheet. Lightly coat the dates with cooking spray. Bake 10 to 12 minutes, until the bacon is crisp. Remove from the oven and set aside. Dot each of the endive leaves with 1 teaspoon of the sour cream. Press the wrapped dates onto the sour-cream-coated endive leaves and serve immediately.

Per serving (2 dates): 251 calories, 17 g protein, 23 g carbohydrates, 12.6 g fat (1 g saturated), 50 mg cholesterol, 4 g fiber, 14 mg sodium

Creamy Mexican Bean Dip with Whole Grain Tortilla Chips

SERVES 8

In my college days, I could eat a whole container of dip with a large bag of greasy potato chips and call that dinner. I didn't realize that I was getting two-thirds of my daily calories and 100 percent of my fat intake for the day with that one indulgence—and I had already eaten breakfast and lunch. This low-fat dip with high-fiber beans is creamy like onion dip and hits the spot, but it also has the vitamin power of spinach.

2	cups baby spinach leaves
2	15-ounce cans low-sodium black beans, drained and rinsed
1	1¼-ounce packet low-sodium taco seasoning without MSG
¼	cup shredded part-skim mozzarella cheese
¼	cup fat-free sour cream
1	2¼-ounce can sliced olives
3	medium tomatoes, chopped
4	romaine lettuce leaves, thinly sliced
1	90-ounce bag whole grain tortilla chips

Preheat the oven to 350°F. Pulse the spinach, beans, and seasoning in a food processor 9 or 10 times, until the beans are smooth and the spinach finely chopped. Transfer to an 8 x 8-inch glass baking dish. Sprinkle with cheese. Bake uncovered 10 to 15 minutes, until the cheese is melted and the bean mixture is warm.

Cool slightly. Using a rubber spatula, smooth the sour cream over the top of the bean mixture. Sprinkle with the olives, tomatoes, and lettuce. Serve immediately with the chips.

Per serving (1 cup dip + ½ cup chips):
187 calories, 7 g protein, 25 g carbohydrates, 7.6 g fat (0.6 g saturated), 1 mg cholesterol, 6 g fiber, 390 mg sodium

Skinny Secret

Who says party food has to be bad for you? A lot of dips and sauces can be perfect places for healthy ingredients, including low-fat dairy.

Nachos Grande with Pickled Jalapeño Salsa

SERVES 6

I could literally eat a plate of nachos as my dinner, so that's what inspired me to create this lower-fat version that is bursting with veggies like broccoli and spinach but still has all those festive Mexican flavors.

- 1 large carrot, peeled and cut into 3 pieces
- ½ small head of broccoli (about ½ pound)
- 2 garlic cloves, chopped
- 1 small hot chile pepper such as jalapeño or serrano, cut into thirds (optional)
- 1 tablespoon olive oil
- 1 pound ground turkey
- 1 1¼-ounce packet low-sodium taco seasoning without MSG
- 1 star anise pod
- 1 cup reduced-sodium chicken or beef broth
- 1 15-ounce can no-salt-added beans, such as black or kidney, drained and rinsed
- 2 cups whole grain tortilla chips
- ¼ cup fat-free sour cream
- 1 cup shredded part-skim mozzarella cheese

SALSA

- ½ cup baby spinach
- ½ ripe Hass avocado, peeled (about ½ cup)
- ¼ cup pickled jalapeño peppers
- ¼ cup cilantro, finely chopped
- 1 lime, zested and juiced
- 1 garlic clove, peeled and cut in half
- ¼ teaspoon salt

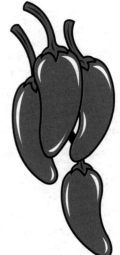

Preheat the oven to 400°F. Line a large baking tray with sides with a piece of aluminum foil. Set aside.

Place the carrot, broccoli, garlic, and chile, if using, in a food processor. Pulse 5 or 6 times, until the vegetables are chopped. Heat a large skillet over high heat. Add the olive oil, chopped vegetables, and turkey. Cook 5 to 6 minutes, breaking up the turkey meat with a spoon. Add the taco seasoning and star anise. Cook 4 to 5 additional minutes, continuing to break up the turkey meat. Add the broth and beans and reduce the heat to medium low. Simmer 5 to 10 minutes, until the meat is cooked through and no longer pink.

Spread the tortilla chips on the baking tray. Spoon the meat mixture over the chips and dot with the sour cream. Sprinkle with cheese. Bake uncovered 10 to 15 minutes, until the cheese is melted and the chips start to brown around the edges.

Meanwhile, place the spinach, avocado, jalapeño, cilantro, lime zest, lime juice, garlic, and salt in a food processor. Pulse until a chunky salsa forms. Serve immediately with the nachos.

Per serving (½ cup chips + 1 cup topping, including salsa): 344 calories, 25 g protein, 22 g carbohydrates, 20.2 g fat (5 g saturated), 75 mg cholesterol, 6 g fiber, 720 mg sodium

Skinny Secret

Poor choice of ingredients makes junk food what it is: junk. Planning ahead and using good starting materials can let you enjoy your favorite comfort foods guilt free.

Hot "Wings" with Spicy Sauce

SERVES 6

I also call these my Better Buffalo Wings and serve them at my monthly ladies' meeting. My friends go crazy for the sauce and don't seem to miss the greasy chicken skin found on traditional hot wings. If you like your sauce "atomic" hot, include the cayenne.

1	15-ounce can reduced-sodium, fat-free beef broth
¼	cup hot sauce, like Tabasco
2	tablespoons no-salt-added tomato paste
2	tablespoons butter
1	teaspoon ground cayenne pepper (optional)
3	pounds skinless, boneless chicken breast, cut into 1-inch-thick tenders
24	12-inch-long wooden skewers
6	celery stalks, trimmed and cut into thirds

First, prepare the dipping sauce: In a small saucepan, stir together the beef broth, hot sauce, tomato paste, butter, and cayenne, if using. Bring to a slow simmer and cook 20 to 25 minutes, until the mixture reduces to about 1 cup.

Skinny Secret

A lot of bar food like hot wings and nachos is invariably hard on the stomach and digestion. Making lighter versions at home will let you enjoy the flavors without a midnight tummy ache.

Thread the chicken onto the skewers. Heat a grill over high heat and cook the skewers 8 to 10 minutes, turning once, until the chicken is cooked through. Drizzle sauce over the skewers and serve the extra sauce on the side with the celery.

Per serving (4 skewers + ⅙ cup sauce): 300 calories, 54 g protein, 2 g carbohydrates, 6.8 g fat (3.2 g saturated), 142 mg cholesterol, 1 g fiber, 404 mg sodium

Party Dip Served with Whole Wheat Pita

SERVES 8, MAKES 4 CUPS OF DIP

When I was a teenager, I used to think this dip in a bread bowl was novel and cute. This grown-up version has a lot more veggies and is served with crusty whole wheat pita—instead of the traditional sourdough bowl that would add a lot of empty calories.

¼ cup light mayonnaise

¼ cup freshly grated horseradish

¼ cup grated Parmesan cheese

2 tablespoons ground flaxseed

2 garlic cloves, mashed

½ teaspoon paprika, plus more for garnish

1 15-ounce can low-sodium white beans, such as navy or cannellini, well drained and rinsed

1 15-ounce can artichoke, drained, rinsed, and chopped

2 cups baby spinach, thinly sliced

¾ cup fat-free Greek yogurt

½ teaspoon salt

¼ teaspoon freshly ground black pepper

4 small whole wheat or whole grain pitas, split in half

2 large celery stalks, cut into matchsticks

2 large carrots, peeled, cut into matchsticks

Preheat the oven to 400°F. In a large bowl, mash the mayonnaise, horseradish, Parmesan, flaxseed, garlic, and paprika to form a smooth paste. Mash the beans until they begin to break apart but are still chunky. Add the beans, artichoke, spinach, yogurt, salt, and pepper to the mayo mixture and stir until well combined.

Transfer the mixture to an 8 x 8-inch or 1-quart baking dish. Smooth the top and sprinkle with paprika. Bake uncovered 10 to 15 minutes, until hot. During the last 5 minutes, spread the pita out directly on the oven rack. Make two stacks of four split pitas each and cut into eight wedges. Serve immediately with dip and vegetable sticks.

Per serving (½ cup): 162 calories, 8 g protein, 22 g carbohydrates, 4.6 g fat (1 g saturated), 5 mg cholesterol, 5 g fiber, 464 mg sodium

Party Mix with Spiced Nuts and Whole Grain Cereal

MAKES 8 CUPS OF PARTY MIX

Don't give up your treats; be a smarter snacker instead. This party mix has a light, salty, spicy zing but is also high in nutrients and whole grain crunch. You won't feel bad sharing this snack with the family since it's low in saturated fat and has a whole lotta fiber going on! Baked chickpeas are the secret ingredient that adds protein and fiber with very little fat.

1	15-ounce can no-salt-added chickpeas, drained and rinsed
	Nonstick cooking spray
¼	teaspoon salt
¼	cup trans-fat-free margarine, melted
2	tablespoons Worcestershire sauce
1	tablespoon reduced-sodium soy sauce
1	teaspoon garlic or seasoned salt
1	teaspoon mild chili powder
1	teaspoon ground cumin
½	teaspoon onion powder
2	tablespoons wheat germ or ground flaxseed
3	cups whole wheat or bran cereal, such as Chex
2	cups whole grain oat cereal, such as Cheerios
1	cup whole wheat pretzel rods
½	cup whole almonds or pecans
½	cup dry roasted peas or soybeans
¼	cup pumpkin seeds

Preheat the oven to 400°F. Line two baking trays with sides with aluminum foil. Turn the chickpeas onto a dish towel or paper towels to dry. Transfer the chickpeas to one of the baking trays and coat with a thin layer of the cooking spray. Sprinkle with the salt and bake 45 to 50 minutes, until the beans become firm and dry.

Meanwhile, combine the remaining ingredients in a large bowl; mix well to coat. Transfer the mix to the second baking tray and bake 5 to 10 minutes, stirring once, until the cereal is crispy and the spices become fragrant.

Cool the beans and cereal mix completely on their trays. Once cool, combine them and store in an airtight container for up to 1 week.

Per serving (½ cup): 167 calories, 6 g protein, 22 g carbohydrates, 7 g fat (1.2 g saturated), 0 mg cholesterol, 4 g fiber, 318 mg sodium

Skinny Secret

Diets don't work when you have to eat foods you don't love: The trick is to make your favorites healthier and your healthier foods tastier.

Main Courses

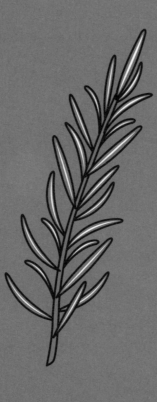

51 CUT THE FAT, KEEP THE CREAMY PASTA CARBONARA

52 MAC AND CHEESE WITH SHREDDED CHICKEN AND CAULIFLOWER

54 LIGHT LASAGNA MADE WITH TURKEY AND VEGGIES

56 STUFFED SHELLS THAT WON'T LEAVE YOU FEELING STUFFED

57 GOOD LOOKIN' GRILLED CHEESE

58 STUFFED PEPPERS COOKED IN PEPPERONI-FLAVORED TOMATO SAUCE

60 RAINBOW MACARONI SALAD WITH TUNA

61 CAJUN CATFISH IN CORNMEAL BREADING

62 FRENCH TUNA SALAD

64 MOCK CRAB CAKES WITH ZUCCHINI AND TUNA

65 SEVEN-MINUTE SALMON

66 STUFFED CHICKEN PARMESAN

67 MY DAD'S TRIM CHICKEN ENCHILADAS

68 BAKED "DEEP FRIED" CHICKEN WITH CRUNCHY DOUBLE WHOLE GRAIN BREADING

70 CHICKEN "NO POT BELLY" PIE

72 JUST LIKE TAKEOUT SWEET-AND-SOUR CHICKEN

74 SESAME CHICKEN HOLD THE DEEP-FRIED BREADING

76 CHICKEN AND RICE HOT POT

78 CHICKEN PAPRIKASH, CREAMY BUT LIGHT CHICKEN STEW

80 CHICKEN MARSALA WITH MUSHROOMS AND BROCCOLI

82 SUPERMOIST TURKEY BURGERS

84 TANTALIZING TURKEY TACOS WITH STAR ANISE

86 BAKED MEATBALLS WITH ZESTY MARINARA

88 MEATBALL SANDWICHES

90 PIGS IN A BLANKET

92 PORK LO MEIN, HOLD THE GREASE

94 SPICY SLOPPY JOES WITH CARROT AND RED BELL PEPPER

96 STEAK AND POTATOES

98 TENDER BEEF STROGANOFF

Cut the Fat, Keep the Creamy Pasta Carbonara

SERVES 6

Carbonara is traditionally made by tossing the pasta in bacon grease and heavy cream. By making this dish with turkey bacon, fat-free yogurt, and half-and-half, you still get those great carbonara flavors without tons of saturated fat.

Nonfat cooking spray

6 slices of nitrate-free turkey bacon, chopped

4 egg yolks

½ cup plain, fat-free Greek yogurt

½ cup grated Parmesan cheese

½ teaspoon coarsely ground black pepper

2 cups frozen peas

1 16-ounce box pasta, such as brown rice or soft multigrain pasta

2 tablespoons half-and-half

¼ cup fresh basil leaves, torn or thinly sliced

Preheat the oven to 425°F. Coat two large cookie sheets with cooking spray. Spread the turkey bacon on the sheets and bake 15 to 20 minutes, until the bacon is crisp. Set aside. In a medium bowl, whisk the egg yolks, yogurt, Parmesan, and pepper until smooth.

Place the peas in a large colander and set it in the sink. Cook the pasta in a stockpot according to the package instructions; drain the pasta on top of the peas to defrost them. Return the pasta and pea mixture to the stockpot and place it over very low heat. Add the egg mixture and turkey bacon. Toss the pasta about 1 minute, until the egg mixture evenly coats the noodles. Turn off the heat, add the half-and-half and stir well. Top with basil and serve immediately.

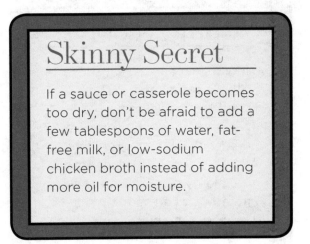

Skinny Secret

If a sauce or casserole becomes too dry, don't be afraid to add a few tablespoons of water, fat-free milk, or low-sodium chicken broth instead of adding more oil for moisture.

Per serving (2 cups): 472 calories, 19 g protein, 66 g carbohydrates, 12 g fat (4 g saturated), 173 mg cholesterol, 4 g fiber, 514 mg sodium

Mac and Cheese with Shredded Chicken and Cauliflower

SERVES 6

Mac and cheese is a staple in many American households, but the box kind has almost no nutritional value. Serve this hearty dish instead. If you want to shorten the recipe preparation time, you can use pregrilled frozen chicken or rotisserie chicken without the skin. You can also buy frozen cauliflower florets, let them defrost on the countertop, and then just stir them in.

- 8 ounces whole wheat or whole brown rice elbow macaroni or penne
  Nonstick cooking spray
- 2 cups fresh cauliflower florets
- 2 boneless, skinless chicken breasts (about 10 ounces)
- ½ teaspoon salt
- 1 teaspoon mild chili powder
- ¼ teaspoon garlic powder
- ¼ teaspoon freshly ground black pepper
- 2 tablespoons trans-fat–free margarine
- 2 garlic cloves, minced
- 3 tablespoons whole wheat flour
- ¼ teaspoon freshly ground nutmeg
- 1½ cups fat-free milk
- 3 cups shredded part-skim mozzarella cheese

Skinny Secret

How to feel full and satisfied without overloading? The key is to eat the meals you crave, like mac and cheese, but prepare them with lighter ingredients like low-fat dairy and incorporate plenty of veggies that are grated or diced so that they are barely detectable!

Preheat the oven to 400°F. In a saucepan, cook the pasta 5 minutes less than the package instructions indicate. Drain and set aside.

Coat a large piece of aluminum foil with cooking spray. Wrap the cauliflower in the foil and place the packet directly on the rack inside the oven. Cover a baking sheet with aluminum foil and coat it with cooking spray. Sprinkle the chicken with the salt, chili powder, garlic powder, and pepper. Set the chicken on the baking sheet and lightly coat the top with cooking spray. Bake the chicken and cauliflower 15 to 20 minutes, until the chicken begins to brown and is no longer pink inside. Remove the chicken and cauliflower from the oven; set the cauliflower aside. Shred the chicken thinly and set aside.

In the pot where the pasta was cooked, melt the margarine over medium-low heat, then add the minced garlic, flour, and nutmeg. Mash the flour into the margarine with the back of a wooden spoon and stir until a thick paste begins to form. Continue to cook 2 to 3 minutes, until the paste starts to leave a light coating inside the pan. Gradually add the milk, whisking constantly, until a thick sauce starts to form. Add the mozzarella and stir until it melts. Turn off the heat and add the pasta, chicken, and cauliflower. Serve immediately.

Per serving (2 cups): 400 calories, 33 g protein, 38 g carbohydrates, 13 g fat (7 g saturated), 65 mg cholesterol, 4 g fiber, 642 mg sodium

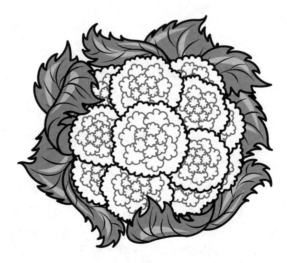

Light Lasagna Made with Turkey and Veggies

SERVES 6 TO 8

Whole wheat lasagna noodles are hard to find but worth the hunt: They are delicious in this recipe. Just boil the noodles first, then drain. Health food stores even sell no-boil whole wheat lasagna noodles that you can simply layer in without precooking. My husband, a confirmed red meat and pasta eater, loves the texture of the ground turkey in the bottom layer, and he never knew—until now!—that the meat was turkey instead of beef.

¼ cup sun-dried tomatoes, chopped

¼ cup boiling water

1 pound ground turkey

1 teaspoon dried oregano

¼ teaspoon salt

¼ teaspoon freshly ground black pepper

   Nonstick cooking spray, preferably olive oil

2 carrots, peeled and grated

¼ cup chopped fresh parsley

2 garlic cloves, minced

2 tablespoons whole wheat flour

1½ cups fat-free milk

1 15-ounce container fat-free ricotta cheese

1 egg white

½ cup grated fresh Parmesan cheese

1 28-ounce can whole tomatoes

1 tablespoon balsamic vinegar

12 cooked whole wheat lasagna noodles

2 cups (8-ounces) shredded part-skim mozzarella

Preheat the oven to 350°F.

Place the tomatoes in the boiling water and set aside. Sprinkle the turkey with the oregano, salt, and pepper. Coat a large skillet with cooking spray and place over high heat. When the skillet is hot, add the turkey, carrots, parsley, and garlic. Cook

2 to 3 minutes, stirring occasionally, until the turkey begins to brown. Spritz the meat (off the heat) with a little more cooking spray if it begins to stick.

Sprinkle the turkey mixture with the flour and reduce the heat to low. Continue to cook, stirring often, until the flour coats the turkey and leaves a light film on the skillet. Add the milk and bring to a slow simmer, stirring occasionally, until a thick sauce forms and the turkey is cooked through.

In a small bowl, stir together the ricotta, egg white, and Parmesan. Set aside. Place the whole tomatoes and sun-dried tomatoes with their liquid in a blender with the balsamic vinegar. Process until smooth. Place 1 cup of the sauce in the bottom of a 9 x 13-inch baking dish. Layer a third of the lasagna noodles on top. Scoop on the turkey mixture. Layer another third of the noodles. Using a rubber spatula, spread on the ricotta mixture and top with the last layer of noodles. Pour the remaining sauce over the lasagna and sprinkle on the mozzarella. Baked uncovered 30 to 35 minutes, until the cheese is bubbly and melted and the filling is hot. Cool 5 minutes, then cut into pieces and serve.

Per serving (2 cups or 1½ cups): 579 calories, 47 g protein, 61 g carbohydrates, 16 g fat (5 g saturated), 72 mg cholesterol, 4 g fiber, 816 mg sodium

Skinny Secret

Struggling with weight? The secret is to focus more—not less—on food. Give food preparation a higher priority in your life, and you'll find that you will enjoy your food rather than eat mindlessly.

Stuffed Shells That Won't Leave You Feeling Stuffed

SERVES 6

Growing up in Pittsburgh, my family ate a lot of rich, heavy American-Italian food. These stuffed shells look like the real deal but have a lot less fat and calories. I tuck in fresh spinach to make this a one-pot meal that makes sense nutritionally when served with a small salad.

- 1 12-ounce box pasta shells
- 2 cups part-skim ricotta cheese
- 2 cups baby spinach, chopped
- 2 egg whites
- ¼ cup grated Parmesan cheese
- 1 28-ounce can whole peeled tomatoes
- 1 teaspoon olive oil
- 2 cloves garlic, chopped
- 1 teaspoon balsamic vinegar
- 2 cups shredded part-skim mozzarella cheese

Preheat the oven to 350°F. In a large saucepan, cook the shells 5 minutes less than the package instructions indicate. Drain and set them in a 9 x 13-inch dish, opening side up. Place the ricotta, baby spinach, egg whites, and Parmesan in a large bowl. Stir until the spinach is combined.

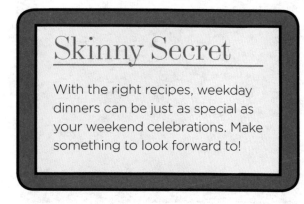

Skinny Secret

With the right recipes, weekday dinners can be just as special as your weekend celebrations. Make something to look forward to!

Spoon the filling into the shells. In a large bowl, place the peeled tomatoes along with their juices, the olive oil, garlic, and balsamic vinegar. Blend with an immersion blender or crush with your hands until a thick sauce forms. Drizzle the sauce over the pasta and top with the mozzarella. Bake uncovered, until the cheese is melted and the filling is hot.

Per serving (2 cups): 531 calories, 35 g protein, 54 g carbohydrates, 18 g fat (10 g saturated), 53 mg cholesterol, 3 g fiber, 762 mg sodium

Good Lookin' Grilled Cheese

SERVES 4

In college, I ate two or three grilled cheese sandwiches for lunch at least 4 days a week. Today, I still love grilled cheese, but just one of these grown-up sandwiches serves as a whole lunch now. As I eat smaller portions, I always include a low-fat protein to help me feel full and add veggies to my lunches and dinners for an extra vitamin boost.

- 4 tablespoons honey mustard
- 8 slices whole wheat or whole grain bread
- 4 slices tomato (about 2 medium tomatoes)
- ½ cup fresh basil leaves
- 4 1-ounce slices nitrate-free deli turkey meat
- 2 cups shredded mozzarella or reduced-fat Swiss cheese
  Nonstick cooking spray
- 8 teaspoons trans-fat-free margarine, softened

Spread the honey mustard on 4 slices of the bread. Place the tomato slices on top, followed by the basil and turkey. Sprinkle on the mozzarella or Swiss cheese. Press the remaining slices of bread on top.

Coat a large skillet or smooth griddle with cooking spray and heat over medium-high heat. Spread half of the margarine on top of the sandwiches. Place the sandwiches margarine side down into the skillet or on the griddle. Spread the remaining margarine on top. Cook 4 to 5 minutes, until the bread is golden and the filling starts to warm. Flip the sandwiches and cook an additional 4 minutes, until the cheese melts. Serve immediately.

Per serving (1 sandwich): 424 calories, 27 g protein, 34 g carbohydrates, 19.7 g fat (5.4 g saturated), 10 mg cholesterol, 5 g fiber, 930 mg sodium

Skinny Secret

Even when you don't crave vegetables, you can find simple ways of tucking them in without detracting from the dish's main flavors.

Stuffed Peppers Cooked in Pepperoni-Flavored Tomato Sauce

SERVES 4

Both hot and mild peppers are easy to find and cook with. I often use them because they heighten flavors in foods as they pack properties with benefits to the body, like vitamin C for skin and gum health, and the powerful anti-inflammatory capsaicin.

- 1 cup short-grain brown rice
- 1 tablespoon olive oil
- 4 pieces of sandwich pepperoni (¾ ounces), chopped
- 3 garlic cloves, crushed or chopped
- 1 tablespoon tomato paste
- 1 26-ounce can whole peeled tomatoes
- ½ cup water
- 1 pound ground turkey
- ½ small onion, chopped
- 1 carrot, chopped or grated
- 1 celery stalk, chopped or grated
- ¼ cup basil leaves, chopped
- 2 egg whites
- ¼ teaspoon salt
- ¼ teaspoon freshly ground black pepper
- 4 green, red, or orange bell peppers

Cook the brown rice according to the package instructions. Drain and place in a large mixing bowl.

Heat the oil in a large stockpot over medium-high heat. Add the pepperoni and garlic. Decrease the heat to medium low and cook 2 to 3 minutes, stirring occasionally, until the garlic becomes fragrant but does not brown. Add the tomato paste and cook 1 to 2 minutes, stirring often, until the paste browns lightly. Add the peeled tomatoes and water. Bring to a slow simmer.

In the same bowl with the rice, place the turkey, onions, carrots, celery, basil, egg whites, salt, and black pepper. Mix with your hands until well combined; the mixture will be wet. Using a small paring knife, cut the tops off the bell peppers. Scoop out the ribs and seeds. Distribute the filling among the peppers and place them in the stockpot with the sauce, filling side up. Cover and simmer 35 to 40 minutes, until the filling is cooked through and the bell peppers are soft. Serve immediately.

Per serving (1 stuffed bell pepper + ½ cup sauce): 498 calories, 29 g protein, 58 g carbohydrates, 17 g fat (4.2 g saturated), 95 mg cholesterol, 8 g fiber, 769 mg sodium

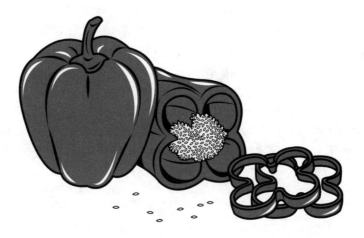

Rainbow Macaroni Salad with Tuna

SERVES 8

Most Americans have a summer food memory that includes macaroni salad. This multicolored version has the same tangy taste but provides protein and loads more veggies so that the salad serves as a complete meal. Leftovers are great to pack for a light lunch.

- ½ cup reduced-fat mayonnaise
- 1 cup plain, fat-free Greek yogurt
- 2 tablespoons cider vinegar
- 2 teaspoons hot sauce, such as Tabasco
- ½ teaspoon salt
- ¼ teaspoon freshly ground black pepper
- 2 cups whole wheat or brown rice pasta, cooked according to the package instructions
- 2 cups broccoli florets, finely chopped
- 1 small red bell pepper, seeded and chopped
- 1 small yellow bell pepper, seeded and chopped
- 1 cup fresh mint leaves, chopped
- 4 hard-boiled eggs, yolks discarded and whites chopped
- 2 jalapeño peppers, seeded and chopped
- 2 celery stalks, chopped
- 2 5-ounce cans tuna packed in spring water, drained

In a large bowl, mix the mayonnaise, yogurt, vinegar, hot sauce, salt, and black pepper until smooth. Toss in the pasta, broccoli, red bell pepper, yellow bell pepper, mint, egg whites, jalapeños, celery, and tuna. Serve immediately or cover and refrigerate for up to 3 days.

Per serving (1½ cups): 217 calories, 16 g protein, 25 g carbohydrates, 6.4 g fat (1.3 g saturated), 17 mg cholesterol, 3 g fiber, 434 mg sodium

Cajun Catfish in Cornmeal Breading

SERVES 4

You can impart flavor from sources beyond salt and fat to create healthy meals that also satisfy. Orange and tomato form a gorgeous flavor combination that I learned about while working in an upscale restaurant in Manhattan. I call this Cajun Catfish because it is spicy, yet it incorporates the sweetness of orange.

- ¼ cup white whole wheat flour or whole wheat pastry flour
- ¼ cup finely ground cornmeal
- 2 tablespoons tomato paste
- 1 large orange, zested and juiced
- 2 tablespoons hot sauce, such as Tabasco
- 4 6-ounce catfish fillets, or other firm white fish like tilapia
- ½ teaspoon salt
- ½ teaspoon ground cayenne pepper
- ½ teaspoon freshly ground black pepper
- 2 tablespoons olive oil
  Nonstick cooking spray

Combine the flour and cornmeal on a piece of waxed paper. Place the tomato paste, orange zest and juice, and hot sauce in a shallow bowl. Sprinkle the fish with the salt, cayenne, and black pepper and dip in the tomato mixture, then dredge in the flour mixture.

Preheat the oven to 400°F. Heat the oil in a large skillet over medium-high heat. Add the fish and cook 3 to 4 minutes. Coat the tops with a layer of cooking spray and turn. Cook 1 to 2 minutes, then bake in oven. Bake 4 to 5 minutes, until the fish flakes when pressed with a fork. Serve immediately.

Per serving (1 piece): 343 calories, 29 g protein, 19 g carbohydrates, 16.8 g fat (3.5 g saturated), 80 mg cholesterol, 4 g fiber, 390 mg sodium

Skinny Secret

Even if you don't like spicy foods, adding a pinch of cayenne or chile flakes can add dimension and warmth to simple dishes—yet you won't break a sweat.

French Tuna Salad

SERVES 4

When I was in college, I had real French food for the first time in Paris, and I noticed that the French could make a salad their entire meal. I was impressed by the amount of vegetables they ate with every meal—at least two or three servings.

DRESSING

¼ cup fat-free sour cream

¼ cup fresh parsley leaves

2 tablespoons red wine vinegar

2 tablespoons water

2 tablespoons lemon juice (about ½ lemon)

2 tablespoons olive oil

2 garlic cloves, peeled and cut into thirds

2 teaspoons Dijon mustard

SALAD

½ pound prewashed mixed greens or 1 large head romaine lettuce, thinly sliced

½ cup quinoa, cooked according to the package instructions

6 small red potatoes, cut in half

1 pound green beans, trimmed and cut into 1-inch pieces

6 tomato wedges

3 hard-boiled eggs, yolks discarded and whites chopped

½ cup pitted black olives

1 6-ounce can light tuna packed in spring water, drained

1 small Hass avocado, peeled and cubed

2 ounces fresh mozzarella cheese, cubed (about ½ cup)

½ red onion, thinly sliced

Place the sour cream, parsley, vinegar, water, lemon juice, oil, garlic, and mustard in a minichopper. Process until smooth. Set aside.

Arrange the mixed greens or lettuce on a large platter. Sprinkle the quinoa over the greens.

Place the potatoes in small saucepan and cover with water. Bring to a boil and cook uncovered 15 to 20 minutes, until tender. Add the green beans during the last 5 minutes of cooking. Drain the potatoes and beans.

Arrange the potatoes, beans, tomatoes, egg whites, olives, tuna, avocado, and mozzarella on top of the greens. Top with the red onion and drizzle with the dressing. Serve immediately.

Per serving (2 cups salad + 2 tablespoons dressing): 361 calories, 21 g protein, 33 g carbohydrates, 18 g fat (4 g saturated), 22 mg cholesterol, 10 g fiber, 364 mg sodium

Note: Quinoa is an amazing, fast-cooking soft whole grain. Kids love it because it looks like minipasta, but I love it since it's full of manganese to relax blood vessels for heart health and iron to transport oxygen throughout the body.

Skinny Secret

Most diets force radical changes rather than gently transitioning your stomach to smaller portion sizes. Increase the amount of fiber and low-fat protein to make the change easier.

Mock Crab Cakes with Zucchini and Tuna

SERVES 4

Crab is delicious but can be costly and hard to find in some supermarkets. This version uses easy-to-find tuna. This dish makes a good burger substitute for vegetarians who eat fish.

2	slices whole wheat bread
½	cup plain, fat-free Greek yogurt
¼	cup reduced-fat mayonnaise
1	egg white
1	teaspoon Dijon mustard
1	teaspoon reduced-sodium soy sauce
2	dashes of hot sauce, such as Tabasco
½	teaspoon paprika
½	teaspoon salt
1	large zucchini, grated
1	cup baby spinach, finely sliced or chopped
1	celery stalk, chopped
1	5-ounce can light tuna packed in spring water, drained
1	tablespoon olive oil

Place the bread in a food processor. Pulse 4 or 5 times, until coarse bread crumbs form. Transfer the crumbs to a sheet of waxed paper. Set aside.

In a large bowl, mix the yogurt, mayonnaise, egg white, mustard, soy sauce, hot sauce, paprika, and salt together until smooth. Add the zucchini, spinach, celery, and tuna; stir until well combined. The mixture will be moist. Form the mixture into eight 4-inch-wide patties and place on a plate or sheet of waxed paper. Dip the cakes in the bread crumbs.

Heat the oil a large skillet over medium-high heat. Add the cakes, leaving about 1 inch between each. Cook 4 to 5 minutes per side, turning once, until both sides are crisp and browned. Serve immediately.

Per serving (2 patties): 186 calories, 14 g protein, 12 g carbohydrates, 9.3 g fat (1.7 g saturated), 14 mg cholesterol, 2 g fiber, 702 mg sodium

Seven-Minute Salmon

SERVES 4

Most people who love Asian flavors will adore this dish, especially if it is served alongside Simple Sautéed Spinach with Garlic and Chile Flakes (page 122). The topping is a cross between a peanut sauce and teriyaki. Fish can make a healthy, satisfying meal, and this recipe is so simple that even a beginner home cook who is intimidated by cooking fish can make it with ease.

    2 small limes, zested and juiced
    3 tablespoons reduced-fat peanut butter
    3 tablespoons reduced-sodium soy sauce
    1 1-inch piece fresh ginger, peeled and chopped
    2 garlic cloves, chopped
       Nonstick cooking spray
    4 6-ounce boneless wild salmon fillets, skin on

Preheat the oven to 425°F. In a small bowl, mix the lime zest, lime juice, peanut butter, soy sauce, ginger, and garlic. Heat a large skillet over high heat. Coat the skillet with cooking spray and place the salmon fillets in the pan, flesh side down. Cook 1 to 2 minutes, until the salmon starts to brown. Turn the fillets over and turn off the heat. Spoon the lime mixture over the salmon and slide the skillet into the oven. Bake 7 to 8 minutes, until the salmon flakes when pressed with a fork.

Per serving (1 piece): 334 calories, 38 g protein, 11 g carbohydrates, 15.3 g fat (2.6 g saturated), 94 mg cholesterol, 2 g fiber, 600 mg sodium

Skinny Secret

Part of integrating eating healthier habits into a busy lifestyle is choosing ingredients that you can prepare in minutes. Fish fits the bill perfectly.

Stuffed Chicken Parmesan

SERVES 4

I love breaded chicken, and this version has a surprise inside—melted cheese! As a private chef, I used to make this lighter version for my clients all the time. Serve with veggies or a side salad topped with fresh lemon for a complete, healthy meal.

    Nonstick cooking spray
  2 egg whites
 ½ cup prepared pasta sauce
  2 cups whole wheat bread crumbs
  1 tablespoon fresh parsley, chopped
 ¼ teaspoon freshly ground black pepper
  4 boneless, skinless chicken breasts (about 1½ pounds)
 ½ cup shredded part-skim mozzarella cheese

Preheat the oven to 400°F. Line two baking sheets with aluminum foil and coat with cooking spray. Set aside.

Whisk the egg whites and pasta sauce in a shallow dish until well combined. Place the bread crumbs, parsley, and pepper on a sheet of waxed paper. Mix well with your fingertips until the parsley is well combined with the bread crumbs. Make a slit in the side of each chicken breast and tuck in 2 tablespoons of the mozzarella. Slice the breasts against the grain into fingers about 1 inch thick. Dip each finger into the sauce mixture and then press into the bread crumbs.

Skinny Secret

Because healthy dishes have less fat, they can dry out easily. Baking provides a more gentle heat that helps ensure chicken, fish, and filet mignon retain their moisture.

Transfer the chicken fingers to the baking sheets and coat with a thick layer of cooking spray. Bake 20 to 25 minutes, until the chicken has lightly brown and is cooked through. Serve immediately.

Per serving (1 piece): 289 calories, 46 g protein, 14 g carbohydrates, 4 g fat (1 g saturated), 99 mg cholesterol, 3 g fiber, 433 mg sodium

My Dad's Trim
Chicken Enchiladas, page 67

Stuffed Shells That Won't
Leave You Feeling Stuffed, page 56

My Dad's Trim Chicken Enchiladas

SERVES 8

My dad is a fantastic cook who loves Mexican food—though he's not used to cooking with a lot of Mexican ingredients. He uses Italian ingredients, such as ricotta cheese. If you like hot and spicy food like I do, add 1 teaspoon of ground cayenne pepper to the enchilada sauce.

1 tablespoon olive oil

1 10-ounce package mushrooms, sliced

1 red bell pepper, seeded and chopped

½ Vidalia or yellow onion, diced

1 teaspoon fresh thyme leaves

1 teaspoon fresh rosemary leaves, chopped

½ teaspoon salt

2 boneless, skinless chicken breasts (about ¾ pound), cut into 1-inch chunks

½ teaspoon mild chili powder

1 cup part-skim ricotta cheese

1 10-ounce can enchilada sauce

8 small (8-inch) fajita-size whole wheat or whole grain flour tortillas

2 cups shredded part-skim mozzarella cheese

Preheat oven to 400°F. Warm the oil in a large skillet over high heat. Add the mushrooms, peppers, onions, thyme, rosemary, and salt. Cook 8 to 10 minutes, until softened. Transfer to a plate. Sprinkle the chicken with chili powder. Increase the skillet heat to high and add the chicken. Cook 5 to 6 minutes, until the chicken starts to brown. Turn the heat off and stir in the ricotta and vegetables.

Place the enchilada sauce in a shallow dish. Warm the tortillas in the oven in a single layer 4 to 5 minutes. Remove from the oven and lightly coat each with the enchilada sauce. Put scoops of the chicken mix on top of the tortillas, followed by sprinkles of cheese. Fold the tortillas over the filling and roll up like a cigar. Using a spatula, place the tortillas in the baking dish. Repeat the process with all the tortillas. Pour any remaining sauce over the rolled tortillas and top with the remaining cheese. Bake uncovered for about 20 minutes, until the enchiladas are bubbly and cracked on top.

Per serving (1 enchilada + ¼ cup sauce): 253 calories, 22 g protein, 20 g carbohydrates, 11 g fat (3.4 g saturated), 30 mg cholesterol, 2 g fiber, 572 mg sodium

Baked "Deep Fried" Chicken with Crunchy Double Whole Grain Breading

SERVES 8

My neighbor's little boy calls this Funky Chicken because the crust looks so interesting. I like this dish because it's healthy, but it's also fit for a large appetite.

Nonstick cooking spray

1½ cups crisp brown rice cereal

½ cup whole wheat bread crumbs

1 tablespoon grated Parmesan cheese

1 tablespoon chopped fresh parsley

1 teaspoon garlic powder

½ teaspoon paprika

¼ teaspoon freshly ground black pepper

¼ teaspoon cayenne pepper

2 eggs

2 egg whites

2 tablespoons honey mustard

8 boneless, skinless chicken breasts (about 3 pounds)

½ teaspoon salt

½ cup whole wheat flour

Preheat the oven to 425°F. Coat two large cookie sheets with cooking spray. Place the rice cereal, bread crumbs, Parmesan, parsley, garlic powder, paprika, black pepper, and cayenne on a large sheet of waxed paper; mix with your fingertips until the spices are well blended.

Place the eggs, egg whites, and honey mustard in a shallow bowl. Whisk until smooth. Sprinkle the chicken with salt and dredge in the flour to coat. Dip each chicken piece in the egg mixture and then dredge in the bread crumbs to coat evenly. Transfer the chicken to the cookie sheets and coat with an even layer of cooking spray. Bake 25 to 30 minutes, until the coating is crisp and the meat is no longer pink in the center. Serve immediately.

Per serving (1 piece): 256 calories, 37 g protein, 17 g carbohydrates, 3.7 g fat (1 g saturated), 136 mg cholesterol, 2 g fiber, 297 mg sodium

Skinny Secret

Fried food has a bad reputation for a very good reason, but you don't have to miss out on that satisfying crunch. Baking "faux" fried foods in the oven is a lot less messy than turning on the fryer, and it's a whole lot better for you.

Chicken "No Pot Belly" Pie

SERVES 4

Creamy chicken potpie filling is so comforting; unfortunately, it's usually made with heavy cream. I've created this lighter version that also provides a light, crunchy topping—minus all the butter.

1 tablespoon olive oil

¼ head cauliflower, cut into florets

2 carrots, peeled and chopped

2 celery stalks, chopped

½ red or yellow onion, chopped

2 boneless, skinless chicken breasts (about ¾ pound), cut into 2-inch cubes

2 tablespoons all-purpose flour

½ teaspoon salt

½ teaspoon mild chili powder

¼ teaspoon freshly ground black pepper

¼ teaspoon paprika

1½ cups fat-free milk

1 cup frozen peas

2 tablespoons reduced-fat mayonnaise

1 teaspoon Dijon mustard

4 large sheets of phyllo

Nonstick cooking spray

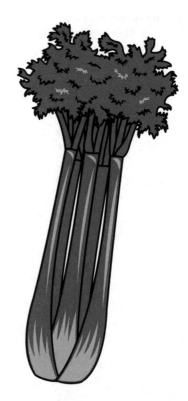

Preheat the oven to 350°F. Heat the oil in a large skillet over medium-high heat. Add the cauliflower, carrots, celery, and onions. Cook 8 to 10 minutes, until the vegetables soften. Sprinkle the chicken with the flour, salt, chili powder, pepper, and paprika. Add the chicken to the skillet. Cook 2 to 3 minutes, stirring once or twice, until the chicken just starts to brown and is cooked through.

Add the milk to the skillet and bring it to a boil, stirring often, until a thick sauce forms. Add the peas, mayonnaise, and mustard. Simmer 5 to 10 minutes, until the cauliflower is tender. Transfer the chicken mixture to four ovenproof bowls. Coat each sheet of phyllo with cooking spray and stack the sheets on top of each other. Cut the stack into four pieces and press each piece on top of each bowl. Bake the potpies 10 minutes, until the phyllo is crisp. Serve immediately.

Per serving (1½ cups): 298 calories, 25 g protein, 30 g carbohydrates, 8.3 g fat (1.6 g saturated), 45 mg cholesterol, 4 g fiber, 656 mg sodium

Skinny Secret

Phyllo is paper-thin sheets of unleavened flour dough used for making flaky pies and pastries. You'll find it fresh or frozen in the grocery store.

Just Like Takeout Sweet-and-Sour Chicken

SERVES 8

I love the way this chicken dish looks like the real deal. But it's so much lighter on the oil compared to the fat that typically coats the inside of a take-out carton. I sweeten this dish with orange juice instead of sugar for an extra boost of vitamin C.

SAUCE

- 1 cup orange juice
- 4 garlic cloves, minced
- 1 lemon, juiced
- 1 tablespoon orange marmalade
- 1 tablespoon cornstarch
- 1 tablespoon sesame oil

CHICKEN

- Nonstick cooking spray
- ½ cup whole wheat flour
- 2 tablespoons fine cornmeal
- 1 tablespoon cornstarch
- 2 egg whites
- 2 boneless, skinless chicken breasts (about ¾ pound), cut into 1-inch cubes
- ½ teaspoon salt
- ¼ teaspoon paprika
- 1 red bell pepper, seeded and chopped
- 1 yellow or green bell pepper, seeded and chopped
- 1 cup broccoli florets
- 1 red onion, cubed
- ½ cup cubed pineapple
- 1 8-ounce can bamboo shoots, drained
- 1 cup short-grain brown rice, cooked according to the package instructions

Place the orange juice, garlic, lemon juice, marmalade, cornstarch, and sesame oil in a large bowl and whisk until smooth.

Preheat the oven to 450°F. Coat a large cookie sheet with cooking spray. Place the flour, cornmeal, and cornstarch on a large sheet of waxed paper. Mix with your fingertips until the cornmeal is well incorporated. Place the egg whites in a shallow bowl. Sprinkle the chicken with salt and paprika. Dip the chicken cubes in the egg whites and then in the flour-cornmeal mixture. Place the chicken chunks 1 inch apart on the cookie sheet. Coat the chicken with a thick layer of the cooking spray. Bake 10 to 15 minutes, turning occasionally, until the chicken is cooked through and the breading is crisp.

Heat a large skillet over high heat. Coat the skillet with cooking spray and add the bell peppers, broccoli, and onions. Cook 4 to 5 minutes, stirring often, until the vegetables start to brown lightly but are still crisp. Stir in the pineapple and bamboo shoots. Transfer the chicken to the skillet with the vegetables. Drizzle with the sauce and gently stir until the sauce coats the chicken. Cook 1 to 2 minutes more, until the sauce thickens. Serve immediately with rice.

Per serving (2 cups with rice): 238 calories, 14 g protein, 39 g carbohydrates, 3 g fat (0.5 g saturated), 21 mg cholesterol, 4 g fiber, 191 mg sodium

Skinny Secret

When you get your mealtime fix from take-out places, it's hard to truly eat healthy: You could get three times your daily amount of fat in just one meal!

Sesame Chicken Hold the Deep-Fried Breading

SERVES 4

I gave this Chinese classic a major facelift. It has that great sesame flavor without the breading, and I boosted the nutrition by adding lots of fresh veggies.

2 boneless, skinless chicken breasts (about ¾ pound), thinly sliced

1 medium orange, zested and juiced

2 tablespoons brown sugar

3 tablespoons reduced-sodium soy sauce

1 1-inch piece of fresh ginger, finely chopped

2 teaspoons hot chile sauce, such as sriracha

1 cup low-sodium chicken broth

1 tablespoon cornstarch

1 tablespoon sesame oil

1 red bell pepper, seeded and cut into 1-inch pieces

1 orange or yellow bell pepper, seeded and cut into 1-inch pieces

1 yellow or red onion, cut into 1-inch pieces

2 cups baby spinach leaves

1 5-ounce can bamboo shoots, drained and rinsed

2 tablespoons toasted sesame seeds

1 cup short-grain brown rice, cooked according to the package instructions

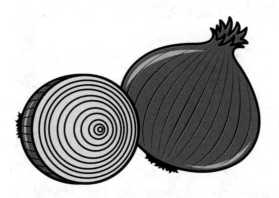

Place the chicken, orange zest, orange juice, brown sugar, soy sauce, ginger, and hot sauce in a medium bowl. Stir well to coat the chicken. Cover and marinate in the refrigerator at least 1 hour or overnight.

Place the broth and the cornstarch in a coffee mug and stir well. Heat a large skillet or wok over high heat for about 1 minute. Add the oil. Carefully add the bell peppers and onions. Cook 2 to 3 minutes, stirring often, until the veggies start to brown lightly. Add the spinach and bamboo shoots and cook 1 to 2 additional minutes, until the spinach begins to wilt.

Transfer the vegetables to a plate. Reduce the heat to medium and add the chicken and marinade to the skillet or wok. Cook 2 to 3 minutes, stirring occasionally, until the chicken begins to cook and the marinade dries up. Return the vegetables to the skillet or wok and add the cornstarch mixture. Stir well and decrease the heat to low. Cook 1 to 2 minutes longer, until the sauce thickens and the chicken is cooked through. Sprinkle with sesame seeds and serve immediately with the rice.

Per serving (½ cup rice + 1½ cups chicken and veggies): 424 calories, 24 g protein, 63 g carbohydrates, 7.4 g fat (1 g saturated), 41 mg cholesterol, 4 g fiber, 572 mg sodium

Skinny Secret

What makes Chinese food so popular? For me, it's more the Asian flavors and sauce than the deep-frying and breading. Cooking with savory spices and sauces can boost flavor and keep you feeling satisfied.

Chicken and Rice Hot Pot

SERVE 4

Chicken can sometimes dry out when cooked, but the chicken in this stew is tender and moist and makes a one-pot meal that's great on a cold winter night. Flavorful olives lend a tang to the sauce; just watch out for the pits that I like to leave in for added moisture.

- 4 skinless chicken breasts on the bone (about 1¼ pounds)
- 1 teaspoon paprika
- 1 teaspoon dried rosemary
- ¼ teaspoon salt
- ¼ teaspoon freshly ground black pepper
- 1 tablespoon olive oil
- 1 1-inch chunk smoked low-sodium deli ham, trimmed and cubed
- 1 red, yellow, or orange bell pepper, seeded and chopped
- ½ cup short-grain brown rice
- 2 garlic cloves, minced
- ½ cup white wine
- 1 28-ounce can low-sodium peeled tomatoes
- ½ cup assorted olives, pits in
- ¼ cup fresh basil leaves, torn or thinly sliced

Preheat the oven to 350°F. Sprinkle the chicken with the paprika, rosemary, salt, and pepper. Heat the oil in a large skillet over high heat. Add the chicken pieces, meat side down; cook 4 to 5 minutes, until the chicken begins to brown. Turn the chicken and sprinkle the ham chunks around. Cook 4 to 5 minutes more, until the underside of the chicken browns. Transfer the chicken to a plate.

Reduce the heat to medium and add the bell peppers, rice, and garlic to the skillet. Cook 2 to 3 minutes, until the garlic is fragrant and the rice picks up some of the oil. Add the wine and bring to a boil. Cook 2 to 3 minutes, until the wine decreases by half. Add the tomatoes and olives. Bring to a boil while breaking up the tomatoes, and return chicken to the skillet. Cover the skillet and slide it into the oven. Bake 35 to 40 minutes, until the chicken is cooked through. Sprinkle with basil and serve immediately.

Per serving (1 piece chicken + 1 cup rice and sauce): 371 calories, 33 g protein, 35 g carbohydrates, 8.5 g fat (1.5 g saturated), 72 mg cholesterol, 5 g fiber, 724 mg sodium

Skinny Secret

The trick to stop hunger in its tracks is to construct well-balanced meals using hunger-busting proteins with little fat, like chicken without the skin, ground turkey, and egg whites.

Chicken Paprikash, Creamy but Light Chicken Stew

SERVES 8

I grew up eating chicken paprikash, watching Granny temper the sour cream so it wouldn't curdle in the hot, savory broth. This version is lighter, but has the flavor burst and characteristic pink hue of the original that I still crave to this day.

½ cup whole wheat flour

3 tablespoons Hungarian paprika

⅛ teaspoon cayenne pepper

4 chicken breasts on the bone (about 1¼ pounds), skin removed and fat trimmed

½ teaspoon salt

¼ teaspoon freshly ground black pepper

1 tablespoon canola oil

1 large onion, chopped

2 celery stalks, chopped

2 cups reduced-sodium, fat-free chicken broth

1 cup reduced-fat sour cream

1 cup short-grain brown rice, cooked according to the package instructions

Skinny Secret

Creamy doesn't have to mean fattening. The soothing, creamy texture of comfort foods can be created with the right low-fat dairy products.

Place the flour, 2 tablespoons paprika, and the cayenne on a large sheet of waxed paper. Mix the paprika into the flour with your fingertips. Sprinkle the chicken with the salt and black pepper. Dredge the chicken pieces in the flour mixture.

Heat the oil over high heat in a large Dutch oven or a large, heavy stockpot. Add the chicken and brown it on both sides, about 10 minutes. Remove the chicken from the pot and set it on a plate. Reduce the heat to medium and add the onions, celery, and remaining 1 tablespoon paprika to the pot. Cook 4 to 5 minutes, until the onions are soft. Return the chicken to the pot and add enough chicken broth to cover.

Bring to boil, reduce heat, and cover. Simmer 20 to 25 minutes, until the chicken is tender and cooked through. Remove the chicken from the liquid and cool slightly, about 5 minutes. With your fingers or a fork, shred the chicken meat. Discard the bones. Place the sour cream in a small bowl or coffee mug and add 1 cup of the stew liquid to it, stirring well. Transfer the sour cream mixture to the pot and add the chicken. Stir well to combine. Serve immediately over the rice.

Per serving (1½ cups stew + ½ cup cooked rice): 257 calories, 19 g protein, 29 g carbohydrates, 7 g fat (2.6 g saturated), 46 mg cholesterol, 3 g fiber, 225 mg sodium

Chicken Marsala with Mushrooms and Broccoli

SERVES 4

This is a great dish for meat lovers. If you can't find thinly sliced chicken cutlets, you can easily make them yourself by cutting skinless, boneless chicken breast lengthwise and pounding the fillets thin with a meat mallet or the back of a heavy ladle.

½ cup whole wheat pastry flour or white whole wheat flour
1 teaspoon paprika
1 teaspoon grated orange zest (from 1 medium orange)
¼ teaspoon freshly ground black pepper
8 thinly sliced chicken breast cutlets (about 1¼ pounds)
½ teaspoon salt
   Nonstick cooking spray
2 tablespoons olive oil
1 10-ounce package mushrooms, such as white button or cremini, sliced
1 shallot or ¼ small red onion, finely chopped
½ cup Marsala wine
1 cup reduced-sodium, fat-free chicken stock
2 cups broccoli florets, roughly chopped
2 tablespoons reduced-fat cream cheese, at room temperature
¼ cup packed flat parsley leaves, chopped

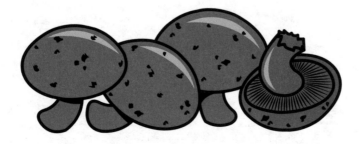

Place the flour, paprika, orange zest, and black pepper on a sheet of waxed paper. Mix with your fingertips until well combined. Sprinkle the chicken with salt and dredge in the flour mixture.

Coat a large skillet with cooking spray. Heat the skillet over medium-high heat and add half of the oil. Shake any excess flour off the chicken and add half of the cutlets to the skillet. Reduce the heat to medium and cook 2 to 3 minutes, until the chicken has a brown crispy coating. Turn once and cook 2 to 3 minutes longer, until chicken is cooked through and no longer pink. Transfer the chicken to a plate. Repeat with the remaining oil and chicken.

Add the mushrooms and shallots or onions to the skillet. Cook 4 to 5 minutes, until the mushrooms soften and begin to brown; add 1 or 2 tablespoons of water if the mushrooms or onions begin to stick. Add the Marsala and bring to a boil, allowing the liquid to decrease by a third. Add the chicken broth and broccoli, then reduce to a simmer and cover. Cook another 4 minutes, until the broccoli is tender. Turn off the heat and slowly add the cream cheese to the skillet, stirring continuously until the cheese starts to combine with the sauce and incorporates the veggies (the stirring keeps the cheese from curdling). Return all the chicken to the skillet. Sprinkle with the parsley and serve immediately.

Per serving (1½ cups): 366 calories, 39 g protein, 21 g carbohydrates, 10.4 g fat (2.2 g saturated), 86 mg cholesterol, 4 g fiber, 549 mg sodium

Skinny Secret

Due to food-safety concerns, most chicken ends up over-cooked, dry, and stringy. Because of its low fat content, chicken should be cooked quickly over high heat. Most skinless, boneless breasts cook in only 4 to 6 minutes!

Supermoist Turkey Burgers

SERVES 4

Cooking meat with vegetables that are high in water content can help keep the meat moist and tender, and the veggies also add a lot of flavor without adding fat. I love hot-and-spicy honey mustard on these burgers. I even eat the leftovers cold, without a bun.

4 teaspoons olive oil
1 10-ounce package mushrooms, finely chopped
½ cup diced red bell pepper
¼ cup finely diced onion
1 garlic clove, minced
½ pound lean ground turkey
¼ cup whole wheat bread crumbs
2 egg whites
¼ cup chopped fresh basil
1 tablespoon reduced-sodium soy sauce
¼ teaspoon freshly ground black pepper
4 whole wheat or whole grain hamburger buns, toasted
4 tablespoons honey or Dijon mustard
1 cup baby spinach leaves, packed

Skinny Secret

Turkey and chicken can be bland. When cooking with low-fat protein, perk up the recipe with fresh herbs and add spices like paprika, garlic powder, and sweet chili powder.

Heat 2 teaspoons of the oil in a large skillet over medium-high heat. Add the mushrooms, bell peppers, onions, and garlic. Cook 5 to 6 minutes, until the vegetables start to soften. Transfer to a large bowl. Add the turkey, bread crumbs, egg, basil, soy sauce, and black pepper.

With your fingertips, stir the mixture until the vegetables are well mixed with the meat. Form four patties 8 inches in diameter. Heat the remaining 2 teaspoons oil in the same skillet over high heat. Add the patties. Reduce the heat to medium and cook 10 to 12 minutes, turning once, until the meat is no longer pink in center.

Transfer the burgers to the buns and top with mustard and spinach leaves. Serve immediately.

Per serving (1 burger): 300 calories, 21 g protein, 27 g carbohydrates, 11.6 g fat (2.5 g saturated), 45 mg cholesterol, 3 g fiber, 788 mg sodium

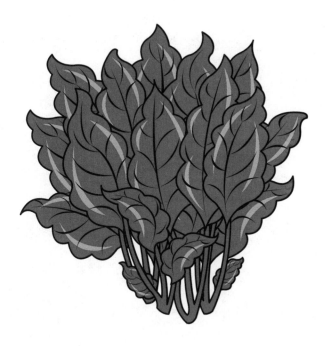

Tantalizing Turkey Tacos with Star Anise

SERVES 4

Since most kids enjoy Mexican takeout, tacos can be a fun family meal. You can feel good about serving this version, which is high in protein and low in fat. The star anise adds sweet flavor and aroma without sugar or fat. You've got to try this dish!

- 1 tablespoon canola oil
- 1 pound lean ground turkey
- 2 teaspoons ground cumin
- 2 teaspoons ground chili powder
- ¼ teaspoon salt
- 1 green bell pepper, finely chopped
- 1 large carrot, grated
- ½ onion, finely chopped
- 2 garlic cloves, minced
- 1 8-ounce can of no-salt-added tomato sauce
- 1 star anise pod
- 1 cup low-sodium canned black beans, rinsed and drained
- 1 cup water
- 1 box taco shells (12 count)
- ½ cup jarred tomato salsa
- 4 large romaine lettuce leaves, thinly sliced
- 2 medium tomatoes, chopped
- ½ cup fat-free sour cream

Heat the oil in a large skillet over high heat. Sprinkle the turkey with the cumin, chili powder, and salt. Add the pepper, carrot, onions, and garlic. Cook 2 to 3 minutes until the pepper starts to soften. Add the turkey meat in one piece and cook 1 to 2 minutes, without stirring until the turkey begins to brown. Cook 7 to 8 minutes, breaking up the meat with a wooden spoon until it is cooked through. Add the tomato sauce and star anise and cook 2 to 3 minutes, stirring occasionally until the mixture is thick. Add the beans and water, then reduce the heat to low. Cook 10 to 15 minutes, until the liquid decreases by half, mashing some of the beans with the back of a spoon. Discard the star anise.

Wrap the taco shells in aluminum foil. Warm the taco shells in a toaster oven for 3 to 4 minutes or in a 350°F preheated oven for 10 minutes. Distribute the turkey mixture evenly among the shells. Top with salsa, lettuce, tomatoes, and sour cream. Serve immediately.

Per serving (2 cups): 463 calories, 37 g protein, 44 g carbohydrates, 17 g fat (3 g saturated), 48 g cholesterol, 7 g fiber, 514 mg sodium

Skinny Secret

I call for romaine lettuce because it's as crunchy as iceberg, plus it contains vitamins A, K, and C. Making small switches can have a huge impact on your overall health.

Baked Meatballs with Zesty Marinara

SERVES 4

Using fresh herbs, like the basil in this dish, is a great way to add interest and flavor without fat or calories. These meatballs are a perfect option for a meat lover who wants a meal that is low in saturated fat. You can serve the meatballs without pasta for a filling meal that is lighter and high in protein.

   Nonstick cooking spray
 1 pound lean ground turkey
 2 cups baby spinach, chopped
 1 cup whole wheat bread crumbs
 ½ cup fat-free milk
 ¼ cup finely grated Parmesan cheese, plus ¼ cup to serve tableside
 2 egg whites
 2 tablespoons fresh basil, thinly sliced
 1 teaspoon garlic powder
 ¼ teaspoon salt
 ¼ teaspoon freshly ground black pepper
 2 tablespoons low-sodium tomato paste
 1 cup white or red wine
 1 26-ounce can whole peeled tomatoes
 2 sprigs fresh basil
 1 teaspoon red pepper flakes
 1 teaspoon dried oregano

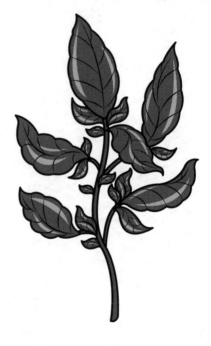

Preheat the oven to 400°F. Coat an 8 x 12-inch baking dish with high sides with cooking spray.

In a large mixing bowl, combine the turkey, spinach, bread crumbs, milk, cheese, egg whites, basil, garlic powder, salt, and black pepper. Using your hands, mix all ingredients until well incorporated. Form into 2-inch balls. Set the meatballs into the prepared baking dish.

Bake the meatballs 20 to 25 minutes, turning once or twice, until well browned. Remove the dish from the oven and slide the meatballs to the side. Add the tomato paste to one corner and pour the wine over the tops of the meatballs. Return the dish to the oven and bake 5 minutes.

Remove the dish again and mix in the tomatoes, basil sprigs, pepper flakes, and oregano. Cover the dish with aluminum foil and bake for an additional 20 minutes, until a sauce forms and the meatballs are cooked through. Serve immediately with grated cheese and pasta or a whole grain baguette.

Per serving (4 meatballs + 1 cup sauce): 352 calories, 29 g protein, 20 g carbohydrates, 11.5 g fat (3.6 g saturated), 94 mg cholesterol, 4 g fiber, 832 mg sodium

Skinny Secret

If you want your children to eat right, pick recipes that are visually appealing to kids—foods like tacos, meatballs, and lasagna.

Meatball Sandwiches

SERVES 8

I still remember the meatball subs my Uncle Jerry used to make when I was a kid. He would serve the savory meatballs on a huge, crusty Italian roll. Now that I'm older and wiser, I still want the sandwich's classic luscious tomato sauce, meat, and cheese, but with more nutrition and less fat.

1 pound lean ground turkey

1 small zucchini, grated

1 large carrot, grated

1 cup whole wheat bread crumbs

½ cup fat-free milk

¼ cup grated Parmesan or Romano cheese

¼ cup fresh parsley or basil leaves, thinly sliced

1 egg

2 garlic cloves, minced

¼ teaspoon salt

¼ teaspoon freshly ground black pepper

Nonstick cooking spray

1 tablespoon olive oil

2 tablespoons tomato paste

1 28-ounce can low-sodium diced tomatoes

½ cup white wine or water

2 20-inch whole grain or whole wheat baguettes, cut into 8 equal pieces, split

1 cup shredded part-skim mozzarella

Place the turkey, zucchini, carrot, bread crumbs, milk, Parmesan or Romano, parsley or basil, egg, garlic, salt, and pepper in a large bowl. Mix the ingredients with your fingers until smooth. Form into about 16 two-inch balls and place on a sheet of waxed paper.

Brown meatballs in two batches. Coat one large skillet with cooking spray. Add half the olive oil and warm over medium-high heat. Add half the meatballs and brown 4 to 5 minutes, carefully turning once. Transfer the meatballs to a plate. Add the rest of the olive oil and the remaining meatballs to the same skillet and brown. Return the first batch of meatballs to the skillet and add the tomato paste. On low heat, cook 1 to 2 minutes without stirring, until the paste starts to brown slightly. Slowly add the diced tomatoes and wine or water. Bring to a slow simmer and cover. Cook 20 to 25 minutes, until the liquid reduces slightly and the meatballs are cooked through.

Preheat the oven to 400°F. Cover a large cookie sheet with aluminum foil. Divide the meatballs among the baguette pieces. Sprinkle the meatballs with the mozzarella. Top with the remaining bread.
Bake for 10 minutes, until the cheese is melted. Serve immediately.

Per serving (1 sandwich): 344 calories, 22 g protein, 36 g carbohydrates, 10 g fat (3.6 g saturated), 83 mg cholesterol, 4 g fiber, 634 mg sodium

Skinny Secret

Having trouble finding whole wheat bread crumbs? Make your own with good quality whole wheat bread. Just pulse it in your food processor. Want a low-sodium tomato sauce? Make your own in the same food processor by selecting low-sodium canned tomatoes, garlic, and onions—and don't forget the fresh basil!

Pigs in a Blanket

SERVES 8

When I was growing up, hearty cabbage-and-tomato Pigs in a Blanket were staples at our family dinner table. Making the simple swap from beef and ground pork to beef and turkey lightens up this dish without drastically changing its flavor.

1	green cabbage head (about 1½ pounds)
½	pound lean ground turkey
½	pound lean ground beef
½	cup short-grain brown rice, cooked according to the package instructions
½	red onion, chopped
2	carrots, peeled and grated or chopped
2	celery stalks, chopped
2	jalapeño peppers, seeded and chopped
1	teaspoon paprika
½	teaspoon salt
¼	teaspoon freshly ground black pepper
1	10-ounce can reduced-sodium tomato soup
2	15-ounce cans no-salt-added diced tomatoes

Skinny Secret

Canned tomatoes are skinny staples in my pantry: They store well, can be used for many recipes, and have little fat. And the low-sodium versions are great for stews and soups.

Bring a large stockpot of water to a boil. With a small paring knife, remove the core of the cabbage. Submerge the cabbage in the water. With a pair of tongs, peel away the outer of leaves of the cabbage and transfer them to a plate. Continue to remove the cabbage leaves, until you have about 16 large leaves. Remove the remaining cabbage, thinly slice it, and discard the water.

With the paring knife, trim off the tough spines of the cabbage leaves. In a large bowl, combine the turkey, beef, rice, onions, carrots, celery, jalapeños, paprika, salt, and black pepper. Mix the ingredients with your hands or a wooden spoon until the veggies and rice are incorporated. Take about ¼ cup of the meat mixture and place it in each cabbage leaf. Roll up the cabbage leaves and tuck in the sides. Transfer the stuffed cabbages to the same stockpot where you boiled the cabbage. Cover the cabbage with the can of tomato soup and both cans of diced tomatoes. Add one can full of water, but do not stir. Cover and bring to boil. Immediately reduce to a simmer. Cook 45 to 50 minutes, covered, until the cabbage is tender and the meat is cooked through. Serve immediately.

Per serving (2 pieces + 2 cups sauce): 199 calories, 17 g protein, 27 g carbohydrates, 2.5 g fat (0.8 g saturated), 28 mg cholesterol, 5 g fiber, 274 mg sodium

Pork Lo Mein, Hold the Grease

SERVES 6

Lo mein is a popular dish packed with thick, tasty noodles. This version is more balanced than what you'll find in a restaurant, since it's a lot lower in fat and has plenty of veggies to boot.

½ cup orange juice (or the juice from 1 orange)

½ cup reduced-sodium, fat-free chicken broth

2 tablespoons reduced-sodium soy sauce

2 tablespoons peanut butter

2 cloves garlic, minced

1 teaspoon red chile flakes or hot chile sauce

1 tablespoon sesame oil

2 center-cut pork chops (about ½ pound), fat trimmed, thinly sliced

1 red bell pepper, seeded and diced

2 cups shiitake mushrooms (about 4 ounces), sliced

1 pound collard greens, thinly sliced

1 8-ounce package soba noodles, cooked according to the package instructions and drained

1 8-ounce can sliced water chestnuts, drained

4 scallions, chopped

In a small bowl, whisk the orange juice, broth, soy sauce, peanut butter, garlic, and red chile flakes or chile sauce until smooth. Set aside. Heat the sesame oil in a large skillet over high heat. Add the pork, bell pepper, shiitakes, and collard greens. Cook 8 to 10 minutes, stirring occasionally, until the vegetables start to soften.

Add the noodles to the skillet with the vegetables. Add the orange juice mixture, water chestnuts, and scallions. Toss well to coat. Cook 1 or 2 additional minutes, until the sauce reduces slightly and the noodles are hot. Serve immediately.

Per serving (1¾ cups): 293 calories, 19 g protein, 43 g carbohydrates, 7.3 g fat (1.4 g saturated), 26 mg cholesterol, 5 g fiber, 606 mg sodium

Skinny Secret

Consistently using too much oil is one of the reasons people have a hard time losing weight. Fat is essential for flavor and taste, but keep a close eye on how much you use.

Spicy Sloppy Joes with Carrot and Red Bell Pepper

SERVES 4

This fresher version of sloppy joes has plenty of veggies to make a portion satisfying without being superhigh in calories. The original version comes from a canned sauce that doesn't have the vitamins or minerals that the veggies provide.

1	small red onion, peeled and cut in half
2	carrots, peeled and cut in thirds
2	celery stalks, cut in thirds
1	red bell pepper, stem removed and seeded
1	tablespoon olive oil
$\frac{1}{2}$	pound lean ground sirloin
2	garlic cloves, cut into pieces
$\frac{1}{4}$	teaspoon salt
1	teaspoon mild chili powder
1	teaspoon ground cumin
1	15-ounce can crushed tomatoes
1	tablespoon tomato paste
1	tablespoon steak sauce
1	tablespoon hot sauce, such as Tabasco
1	teaspoon brown sugar
$\frac{1}{4}$	cup water
4	whole wheat or whole grain hamburger buns

Place the onions, carrots, celery, and bell pepper in a food processor and pulse until finely grated. Heat the olive oil in a large skillet over high heat. Add the grated vegetables, sirloin, garlic, and salt. Cook 7 to 9 minutes, stirring often, until the vegetables soften and the meat begins to cook. Add the chili powder and cumin, cooking 2 to 3 minutes more.

To the skillet add the tomatoes, tomato paste, steak sauce, hot sauce, brown sugar, and water. Bring the mixture to a slow simmer and cook 4 to 5 minutes longer, stirring often, until the mixture is thick and the meat is cooked through. Toast the hamburger buns and spoon out $\frac{1}{2}$ cup of the mixture onto each bun.

Per serving (1 sandwich): 291 calories, 18 g protein, 39 g carbohydrates, 8.2 g fat (1.9 g saturated), 30 mg cholesterol, 8 g fiber, 768 mg sodium

Skinny Secret

Three simple ways to cash in on more veggie nutrition in every meal: Grate, slice, or chop.

Steak and Potatoes

SERVES 4

At every family get-together, my dad tells the story about me as a 4-year-old—you know how parents like to embarrass their kids! We went to a seafood restaurant and I demanded steak, beating my knife and fork on the table and making a huge scene. As an adult, I still love my steak, but I know that eating the right cut of red meat, like lean filet mignon, can mean that we're getting less of the "bad" kind of fat—saturated fat.

2	large baking potatoes, such as Idaho
	Nonstick cooking spray
2	cups reduced-sodium, fat-free beef broth
2	cups dry red wine
4	6-ounce filets mignons, trimmed of excess fat
1/2	teaspoon salt
2	garlic cloves, minced
2	teaspoons freshly cracked assorted peppercorns
2	teaspoons canola oil
2	teaspoons whole wheat flour
2	tablespoons half-and-half
1/4	cup chopped fresh chives or scallions

Preheat the oven to 400°F. Scrub each potato and poke it several times with a fork. Coat the potatoes with cooking spray and bake 50 to 60 minutes, until soft. Place the beef broth and wine in a small saucepan and bring to a simmer; cook 10 to 15 minutes, until the sauce decreases by half.

When the potatoes have baked for about 45 minutes, start the steak. Sprinkle the steaks with salt. Press the garlic and peppercorns onto the steaks. Heat the oil in a large skillet over high heat. When the oil is very hot, carefully add the steaks. Cook the steaks 5 to 6 minutes per side, turning only once, until both sides are well browned. Slide the skillet into the oven and bake 9 to 10 minutes until the center of each steak is still pink but no longer translucent. Remove the steaks to a plate and cover with a piece of aluminum foil (the steak will continue to cook).

Place the skillet over low heat and add the flour to the steak drippings. Cook 2 to 3 minutes, mashing the flour with the back of a wooden spoon until a smooth, thick paste forms. Remove from heat and add the wine sauce. Return the skillet to the burner, whisking the flour mixture for about 1 minute, until a smooth thick sauce forms. Stir in the half-and-half. Serve the sauce over the steaks with half a baked potato per person. Garnish with the chopped chives or scallions and serve immediately.

Per serving (1 steak + ½ potato): 545 calories, 45 g protein, 39 g carbohydrates, 13 g fat (5 g saturated), 117 mg cholesterol, 3 g fiber, 439 mg sodium

Skinny Secret

Why are home-cooked meals more satisfying than takeout? Well, not only does home cookin' make your house smell amazing, but it also enables you to know exactly what's on your plate. In just one take-out meal, you could be getting all the fat and three times the sodium you should consume in one full day.

Tender Beef Stroganoff

SERVES 4

This is a trimmer version of my granny's gorgeous, creamy beef Stroganoff. If you don't have brown rice, try serving this with whole grain angel hair. It also works nicely over Buttermilk Biscuits (page 125).

1	1-pound piece top sirloin, thinly sliced
1	teaspoon mild paprika
½	teaspoon garlic powder
¼	teaspoon freshly ground black pepper
¼	teaspoon salt
2	tablespoons whole wheat flour
1	tablespoon olive oil
1	10-ounce package cremini or button mushrooms, quartered
1	cup reduced-sodium, fat-free beef broth
1	cup water
¼	cup plain, fat-free sour cream
1	head broccoli, cut into 1-inch florets
1	cup short-grain brown rice, cooked according to the package instructions

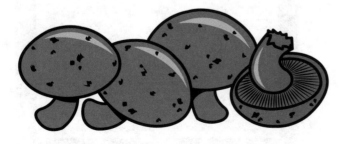

Place the beef on a sheet of waxed paper. Sprinkle it with the paprika, garlic powder, pepper, and salt. Toss the beef to coat. Sprinkle the flour over the beef and turn again until it is entirely coated. Heat the oil in a large pot over medium heat. Shake any excess flour off the beef and add the meat to the pot. Cook 3 to 4 minutes, turning only once or twice, until the beef begins to brown. Add the mushrooms and cook 2 to 3 minutes longer, until the mushrooms start to give off their liquid.

Add the beef broth and water, then bring to a slow simmer and cover. Cook 5 to 10 minutes, until the beef is cooked through but still tender. Remove 1 cup of the liquid and combine with the sour cream. Return to the pot with the beef and stir well to combine.

In a large pot, bring 1 inch of water to a boil. Add the broccoli and cover. Steam 5 to 7 minutes, until the broccoli is tender and still bright green. Serve the beef over the rice and steamed broccoli.

Per serving (2 cups with rice): 427 calories, 36 g protein, 57 g carbohydrates, 8 g fat (2.5 g saturated), 53 mg cholesterol, 8 g fiber, 288 mg sodium

Skinny Secret

To slice beef easily, freeze it for about 30 minutes, until the meat is firm but not rock solid. Slice with a serrated knife.

Light Lasagna Made with Turkey
and Veggies, page 54

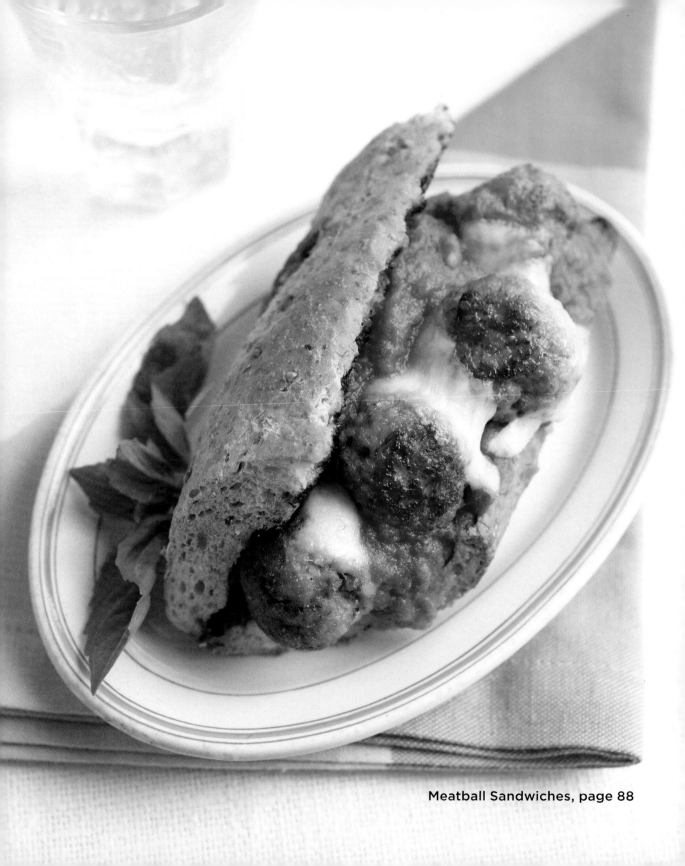

Meatball Sandwiches, page 88

Just Like Takeout
Sweet-and-Sour Chicken, page 72

Steak and Potatoes, page 96

Baked Steak House Fries, page 103

Banana Cream Pie, page 132

Slender Blondie Brownies
with Walnuts, Chocolate Chips, and Prunes, page 146

Southwestern Frittata with
Spicy Corn Salsa, page 8

Frozen Coconut Yogurt, page 159

Tiramisu Parfaits, page 144

Side Dishes

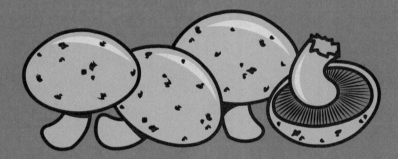

103 BAKED STEAK HOUSE FRIES

104 TWICE-BAKED POTATOES WITH FILLING SO RICH NO ONE WILL KNOW IT'S LOW FAT

105 SCALLOPED POTATOES WITH HAM

107 STUFFED MUSHROOMS WITH BLUE CHEESE

108 BREADED ZUCCHINI WITH MARINARA DIPPING SAUCE

110 SHRIMP AND CORN FRITTERS

112 "MAYONNAISE IS NOT YOUR ENEMY" COLESLAW

113 BROCCOLI BACON SALAD

114 THREE BEAN SALAD

115 CUCUMBER SALAD WITH SOUR CREAM AND FRESH DILL

116 BACON SPINACH SALAD

117 BUTTERMILK YOGURT DRESSING

118 CARROT GINGER DRESSING

119 ALMOND DRESSING

120 GREEN BEANS WITH ALMONDS AND LEMON PEPPER CROUTONS

121 HONEY-ROASTED BABY CARROTS WITH RAISINS

122 SIMPLE SAUTÉED SPINACH WITH GARLIC AND CHILE FLAKES

123 STIR-FRIED GARLIC BROCCOLI

124 WARM CREAMED SPINACH MINUS THE HEAVY CREAM

125 BUTTERMILK BISCUITS

126 WHOLE WHEAT GARLIC BREAD

Baked Steak House Fries

SERVES 4

These fries crisp up nicely in the oven and are best eaten warm, though I must admit I don't mind snacking on the softer, leftover cool fries while I'm making a dinner salad. Keep the potato skins on for extra flavor and fiber.

Nonstick cooking spray

3 large all-purpose potatoes (2 pounds), such as Yukon Gold, cut into 1-inch-thick wedges

3 tablespoons grated Parmesan cheese

1 tablespoon olive oil

½ teaspoon paprika

½ teaspoon mild chili powder

½ teaspoon garlic powder

¼ teaspoon coarsely ground black pepper

½ teaspoon salt

Preheat the oven to 400°F. Cover two cookie sheets with aluminum foil and coat with cooking spray. Place the potato wedges, Parmesan, oil, paprika, chili powder, garlic powder, and pepper in a large bowl, and toss to coat.

Transfer to the baking sheets. Spread the fries out so they are not touching. Bake 20 to 25 minutes, turning once, until the fries are soft in the center and browned on the outside. Sprinkle with salt and serve immediately.

Per serving (½ cup): 216 calories, 6 g protein, 40 g carbohydrates, 4.4 g fat (1 g saturated), 3 mg cholesterol, 3 g fiber, 348 mg sodium

Twice-Baked Potatoes with Filling So Rich No One Will Know It's Low Fat

SERVES 4

When I am in the mood for something creamy and starchy, I like to serve this side dish with a crisp salad.

Nonstick cooking spray
2 large russet potatoes, about 1 pound each
4 slices nitrate-free turkey bacon
1/2 cup reduced-fat sour cream
1/4 cup crumbled Gorgonzola cheese
2 teaspoons hot sauce
1/2 teaspoon salt
1/4 teaspoon freshly ground black pepper
2 scallions, thinly sliced

Preheat the oven to 400°F. Coat a baking sheet with cooking spray. Scrub the potatoes under running water. Poke the potatoes with the tines of a fork. Bake 1 hour, until the potatoes are soft to the touch. Place the bacon on the baking sheet. Slide the tray with the bacon in the oven during the last 15 minutes of baking time for the potatoes. Bake until just crisp. When cool to the touch, roughly chop.

Cut the potatoes in half lengthwise. Scoop out the potato pulp, leaving a 1/2-inch-thick shell, and place the pulp in a large bowl. Add the sour cream, Gorgonzola, hot sauce, salt, and pepper to the pulp. Mash with the back of a fork.

Place the potato skins on a baking sheet. Distribute the mashed filling among the potato skins. Bake 10 to 15 minutes, until the filling is hot. Remove from the oven and sprinkle with the scallions and bacon.

Per serving (1 potato): 283 calories, 13 g protein, 43 g carbohydrates, 7.3 g fat (3.8 g saturated), 43 mg cholesterol, 3 g fiber, 473 mg sodium

Scalloped Potatoes with Ham

SERVES 6

The Japanese mandoline is one of my secret healthy cooking tools; it's inexpensive and a fast way to slice vegetables, even for the beginning cook. For this recipe, I slice the taters superthin so they cook faster and fully capture the flavors of the spices and cheese.

- ¾ pound red potatoes (about 3 medium), well scrubbed
- ¾ pound sweet potatoes (about 1 large), well scrubbed
- 3 tablespoons trans-fat-free margarine
- 3 tablespoons whole wheat flour
- ½ onion, minced
- 4 slices reduced-sodium ham, chopped
- ½ teaspoon freshly grated nutmeg
- ½ teaspoon mild paprika
- ½ teaspoon salt
- ¼ teaspoon freshly ground black pepper
- 1½ cups fat-free milk
- 1¼ cups shredded reduced-fat Swiss cheese
- ¼ cup grated Parmesan cheese

Skinny Secret

A Japanese mandoline might sound like a fancy tool, but it's an inexpensive (and dishwasher safe) vegetable slicer that you can buy online. It is the only slicer you really need in the kitchen.

Continued

Preheat the oven to 400°F. Using a mandoline or a vegetable slicer, slice the potatoes very thin, about $\frac{1}{8}$ inch thick or less, onto a plate or sheet of waxed paper.

Heat the margarine in a large stockpot over medium heat. Add the flour and cook 2 to 3 minutes, mashing the flour into the margarine with the back of a wooden spoon. Add the onions, ham, nutmeg, paprika, salt, and pepper. Cook 1 to 2 minutes longer, until the spices become fragrant.

Increase the heat to high and add $\frac{1}{2}$ cup of the milk, whisking vigorously until a thick paste starts to form. Add the remaining milk and bring to a slow boil, cooking 1 to 2 minutes, until the mixture resembles thick cream. Stir in 1 cup of the Swiss cheese and the Parmesan. Turn the heat off and add the potatoes. Stir well to coat. Transfer the mixture to a 7 x 11-inch baking dish and sprinkle with the remaining $\frac{1}{4}$ cup of Swiss. Bake covered for 20 minutes. Remove the cover and bake an additional 8 to 10 minutes, until the top is browned and the potatoes are cooked through. Serve immediately.

Per serving (1 cup): 256 calories, 16 g protein, 28 g carbohydrates, 10.6 g fat (4.3 g saturated), 20 mg cholesterol, 3 g fiber, 462 mg sodium

Stuffed Mushrooms with Blue Cheese

SERVES 8

Rich, cheesy stuffed mushrooms are a hit at any party, but who says that entertaining has to be unhealthy? I use fat-free sour cream to cut the fat and pick up the flavor of zesty crumbled blue cheese.

- 1 10-ounce package small white button mushrooms
- ¼ cup fat-free sour cream
- ¼ cup crumbled blue cheese
- ¼ cup whole wheat bread crumbs
- 1 teaspoon fresh thyme leaves, chopped
- ½ teaspoon salt
- ¼ teaspoon freshly ground black pepper
- 2 tablespoons fat-free milk
  Nonstick cooking spray
- ½ cup white or rosé wine

Preheat the oven to 350°F. Use a paper towel to wipe any dirt clinging to the mushrooms. Remove the stem from each mushroom. Place half the mushroom stems in a food processor along with the sour cream, blue cheese, bread crumbs, thyme, salt, and pepper, and discard remaining stems. Pulse 4 or 5 times, until the mixture is well blended and slightly chunky. Add the milk and pulse 2 or 3 times, until well mixed.

Place the mushroom caps open side up on a large baking sheet with sides. Spoon the filling into the mushrooms. Coat with a light layer of cooking spray. Pour the wine around the mushrooms. Cover with a large piece of aluminum foil. Bake 15 to 20 minutes, until the mushrooms are tender and the filling is hot. Remove the foil and bake an additional 5 minutes, until the filling begins to brown. Serve immediately.

Per serving (4 mushrooms): 36 calories, 3 g protein, 3 g carbohydrates, 1.5 g fat (1 g saturated), 4 mg cholesterol, 1 g fiber, 222 mg sodium

Breaded Zucchini with Marinara Dipping Sauce

SERVES 4

My granny used to make this from her huge surplus of garden zucchini. It's a tasty way to introduce kids to a juicy, high-fiber vegetable.

1 cup whole wheat bread crumbs

2 tablespoons grated Parmesan cheese

¼ teaspoon garlic powder

¼ teaspoon onion powder

¼ teaspoon dried oregano

¼ teaspoon freshly ground black pepper

2 egg whites

1 tablespoon hot sauce

2 tablespoons whole wheat flour

2 medium zucchinis, sliced into 2 x ½-inch sticks

2 tablespoons olive oil

¼ teaspoon salt

1 cup jarred tomato sauce

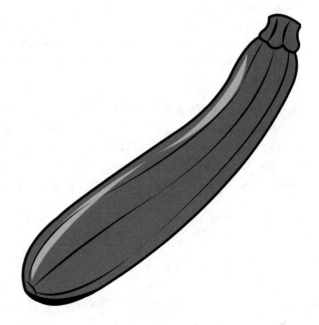

Preheat the oven to 400°F. Place the bread crumbs, Parmesan, garlic powder, onion powder, oregano, and pepper on a sheet of waxed paper. Mix the ingredients with your fingertips until well combined. Set aside. Mix the egg whites and hot sauce in a shallow dish. Place the flour on a sheet of waxed paper. Dip the zucchini in the flour, then in the egg whites, and then in the bread crumb mixture.

Heat two large ovenproof skillets over medium heat. Divide the oil between the two skillets. Add the breaded zucchini and cook 4 to 5 minutes, until the zucchini browns. Turn the zucchini and slide the skillets into the oven. Bake about 10 minutes or until the zucchini is tender. Sprinkle with salt and serve immediately with the sauce.

Per serving (6 sticks): 168 calories, 7 g protein, 18 g carbohydrates, 8.7 g fat (1.8 g saturated), 2 mg cholesterol, 3 g fiber, 565 mg sodium

Skinny Secret

My pantry is stocked with versatile ingredients that can be used in hundreds of recipes—staples like canned tomatoes, low-sodium broth, and whole wheat bread crumbs. Most everything else in my kitchen is fresh, seasonal food.

Shrimp and Corn Fritters

SERVES 4

I started enjoying spicier foods when I was in my twenties, and I found that eating spicy, low-fat foods (including hot chiles) on a regular basis helped curb my cravings for sugar. Not to mention that I was also reaping the heart-healthy benefits from the compounds in chiles.

SWEET CHILE SAUCE

- ¼ cup hot chile sauce, such as sriracha
  Juice of 2 limes
- 2 tablespoons rice wine vinegar
- 2 teaspoons granulated sugar

FRITTERS

- ½ cup white whole wheat flour or whole wheat pastry flour
- 1 teaspoon baking soda
- 1 teaspoon five-spice powder
- ¼ teaspoon salt
- 1 15-ounce can no-salt-added corn, or 2 cups fresh corn kernels (about 5 ears of corn)
- ½ pound raw medium shrimp, shells and tails removed, chopped
- 2 egg whites
- ¼ cup water
- 2 teaspoons freshly grated ginger
- 2 tablespoons canola oil

Preheat the oven to 450°F. In a medium bowl, whisk the chile sauce, lime juice, vinegar, and sugar until smooth. Set aside.

Place the flour, baking soda, five-spice powder, and salt in a large bowl. Stir until the five-spice powder is mixed in well. Add the corn, shrimp, egg whites, water, and ginger. Mix with a wooden spoon until the flour is just combined.

Heat two large ovenproof skillets over medium-high heat. Add 1 tablespoon of the oil to each pan. Drop 2 tablespoons of the fritter batter, 1 inch apart, into the skillets, so that you have six fritters in each pan. Reduce the heat to medium and cook about 2 minutes. Flip the fritters.

Transfer both skillets to the oven and bake 4 to 5 minutes, until the shrimp is cooked through and the batter is no longer wet. Transfer the fritters to a platter and serve immediately with the sauce.

Per serving (3 fritters + 1½ tablespoons of sauce): 302 calories, 18 g protein, 42 g carbohydrates, 8.6 g fat (0.8 g saturated), 86 mg cholesterol, 3 g fiber, 945 mg sodium

Skinny Secret

Sriracha is a Thai version of cocktail sauce that is a lot spicier! Made from sun-ripened chile peppers, vinegar, garlic, sugar, and salt, it bursts with flavor, has only 5 calories per teaspoon, and contains zero fat. Sriracha adds extra dimension to a dish.

"Mayonnaise Is Not Your Enemy" Coleslaw

SERVES 8

I used to think that any dish made with mayonnaise was evil, but I secretly savored mayo's creamy texture and tangy taste. So here's a salad that has the mayo cut with yogurt so you can have the fun and flavor of mayonnaise without the high-fat guilt.

½ cup fat-free Greek yogurt

½ cup reduced-fat mayonnaise

1 tablespoon honey Dijon mustard

1 teaspoon sugar

½ teaspoon celery seeds

½ teaspoon mild chili powder

½ teaspoon paprika

½ teaspoon salt

¼ teaspoon freshly ground black pepper

½ small red cabbage (about ½ pound), cored

1 small fennel bulb, cored

2 carrots, peeled

1 Granny Smith or Gala apple, cored

1 large red onion, thinly sliced

In a large bowl, whisk the yogurt, mayo, mustard, sugar, celery seeds, chili powder, paprika, salt, and pepper until smooth. Using a box grater or food processor, grate the cabbage, fennel, carrots, and apple. Add the grated vegetables along with the onion to the bowl and toss to coat well. Cover and chill at least 1 hour to allow the flavors to combine. Stir well before serving.

Per serving (1 cup): 102 calories, 2 g protein, 12 g carbohydrates, 5.1 g fat (1 g saturated), 5 mg cholesterol, 3 g fiber, 318 mg sodium

Broccoli Bacon Salad

SERVES 8

A salad with bacon and mayo may sound off limits to the health conscious, but thanks to the simple swaps I've made in this recipe, these sinful favorites are no longer forbidden. Fat-free Greek yogurt keeps things creamy without loading on the pounds, and you'll get extra fiber from all the raw veggies.

Nonstick cooking spray

½ pound nitrate-free turkey bacon

½ cup reduced-fat mayonnaise

½ cup fat-free Greek yogurt

2 tablespoons apple cider vinegar

2 tablespoons honey (increase to ¼ cup if more sweetness is desired)

1 head broccoli (about 1½ pounds), cut into very small florets

½ head cauliflower (about 1½ pounds), cut into very small florets

½ cup raisins

½ red onion, minced

Preheat the oven to 400°F. Coat a cookie sheet with cooking spray and spread out the bacon. Bake 10 to 15 minutes, until the bacon is crisp. Set aside.

In a large mixing bowl, whisk the mayonnaise, yogurt, vinegar, and honey until well combined. Chop the bacon. Add the bacon, broccoli, cauliflower, raisins, and onions to the dressing. Toss well to coat. Cover and refrigerate for 1 to 2 hours. Stir before serving.

Per serving (1 cup): 191 calories, 12 g protein, 25 g carbohydrates, 7 g fat (0.8 g saturated), 31 mg cholesterol, 5 g fiber, 180 mg sodium

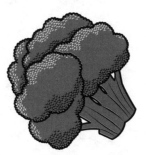

Three Bean Salad

SERVES 8

This summery salad always found its way to my family's picnic tables and summer holiday feasts. This version is a full-flavored alternative to conventional heavy mayonnaise-based macaroni and potato salads.

1 pound green beans, trimmed

1 pound yellow wax beans, trimmed, or one 15-ounce can cut yellow beans, drained and rinsed

6 tablespoons cider vinegar

¼ cup olive oil

¼ cup parsley leaves, chopped

2 tablespoons granulated sugar

1 teaspoon salt

½ teaspoon sweet chili powder

½ teaspoon ground cumin

¼ teaspoon freshly ground black pepper

1 15-ounce can red kidney beans, well drained and rinsed

1 small green bell pepper, seeded and chopped

1 cup sliced red onion

In a stockpot fitted with a steamer basket, bring 1 inch of water to a boil. Steam the green and yellow wax beans for 4 to 5 minutes, until tender crisp. Rinse the beans under cold running water.

In a large mixing bowl, whisk the vinegar, oil, parsley, sugar, salt, chili powder, cumin, and black pepper until smooth. Add the green and yellow wax beans, kidney beans, bell pepper, and onions. Toss well and cover. Chill for at least 4 hours.

Per serving (1 cup): 152 calories, 4 g protein, 20 g carbohydrates, 7 g fat (1 g saturated), 0 mg cholesterol, 7 g fiber, 402 mg sodium

Cucumber Salad with Sour Cream and Fresh Dill

SERVES 4

Cool and crunchy, this salad is a gorgeous accompaniment to something spicy or a great starter to an alfresco lunch. Add 8 ounces cooked shrimp to make it a main course.

1	pound (about 6) small cucumbers, such as Kirby or Persian, peeled and thinly sliced
½	teaspoon salt
½	cup baby spinach leaves, thinly sliced
¼	cup reduced-fat sour cream
2	tablespoons chopped fresh dill
2	teaspoons apple cider vinegar
1	teaspoon granulated sugar
¼	teaspoon ground paprika
¼	teaspoon coarsely ground black pepper

Place the cucumbers in a large colander and sprinkle with half the salt. Let the cucumbers rest for 20 minutes, until they start to give off water. Place the cucumbers on two sheets of paper towel and gently squeeze.

In a medium bowl, place the cucumbers, remaining salt, spinach leaves, sour cream, dill, vinegar, sugar, paprika, and pepper. Stir until the cucumbers are well coated with the sauce. Serve immediately or cover and chill 1 hour before serving.

Per serving (½ cup): 36 calories, 1 g protein, 4 g carbohydrates, 2 g fat (1.1 g saturated), 6 mg cholesterol, 1 g fiber, 309 mg sodium

With shrimp: 103 calories, 15 g protein, 4 g carbohydrates, 3 g fat (1 g saturated), 121 mg cholesterol, 1 g fiber, 471 mg sodium

Bacon Spinach Salad

SERVES 4

I loved this salad growing up because the dressing is hot against cool veggies. Granny made it with ½ pound of high-fat bacon; this leaner version is one you can enjoy without any guilt.

10	ounces baby spinach (about 12 cups)
1	10-ounce package button mushrooms, thinly sliced
4	hard-boiled eggs, yolks discarded and whites chopped
4	6-ounce boneless, skinless chicken breasts
1	teaspoon mild chili powder
½	teaspoon salt
¼	teaspoon freshly ground black pepper
	Nonstick cooking spray
3	teaspoons olive oil
8	slices nitrate-free turkey bacon, thinly sliced
2	large shallots or ½ red onion, minced
¼	cup red wine vinegar
2	teaspoons honey mustard
¼	cup water

Place the spinach, mushrooms, and chopped egg whites in a large bowl. Set aside.

Preheat the oven to 400°F. Sprinkle the chicken with the chili powder, salt, and pepper. Heat a large ovenproof skillet over high heat. Coat the skillet with a thin layer of cooking spray and add 1 teaspoon of the oil. Add the chicken and cook 3 to 4 minutes, until it begins to brown. Turn the chicken, then slide the skillet in the oven and bake 8 to 10 minutes, until the chicken is no longer pink in the center. Remove the chicken from the skillet and let the meat rest 5 minutes before slicing.

Place the skillet that contained the chicken over medium-high heat. Add the remaining oil, bacon, and shallots or red onions. Cook 2 to 3 minutes, until the bacon crisps. Turn the heat off and add the vinegar, honey mustard, and water. Whisk until smooth, pour over the spinach mixture, and toss. Serve immediately.

Per serving (4½ cups): 420 calories, 62 g protein, 13 g carbohydrates, 14.3 g fat (2.8 g saturated), 361 mg cholesterol, 4 g fiber, 601 mg sodium

Buttermilk Yogurt Dressing

MAKES ½ CUP DRESSING

Salads have the reputation for being healthy, but when you drench them in high-fat dressing, you basically cancel out all the health benefits. This dressing is like a rich ranch dressing—minus all the fat!

- ¼ cup low-fat (1 percent) buttermilk
- 1 tablespoon reduced-fat mayonnaise
- 1 tablespoon olive oil
- 6 fresh basil leaves (about 2 tablespoons packed)
- 1 teaspoon Dijon mustard
- ½ garlic clove
- ½ teaspoon mild chili powder
- ¼ teaspoon freshly ground black pepper

Place the buttermilk, mayonnaise, olive oil, basil, mustard, garlic, chili powder, and pepper in a minichopper or blender. Process until smooth. Serve immediately or refrigerate for up to 2 weeks.

Per serving (2 tablespoons): 52 calories, 0 g protein, 2 g carbohydrates, 5 g fat (0.6 g saturated), 2 mg cholesterol, 0 g fiber, 78 mg sodium

Skinny Secret

It's hard to pick out a healthy salad dressing from the multitude of options on store shelves. Making your own dressing takes the guesswork out of deciphering complicated nutrition labels.

Carrot Ginger Dressing

MAKES ½ CUP DRESSING

I love the ginger dressing that comes with a side salad in my local sushi bar, only I don't know what's in the dressing or if the salad is as healthful as it looks. My Carrot Ginger Dressing is very low in fat and a summertime staple in my fridge.

    1 medium carrot, peeled and grated
    1 ½-inch piece of ginger, peeled and grated
  ¼ cup water
    1 tablespoon sesame oil
    1 tablespoon reduced-sodium soy sauce

Place the carrot, ginger, water, oil, and soy sauce in a minichopper or blender. Process until smooth. Serve immediately or refrigerate for up to 4 days.

Per serving (2 tablespoons): 40 calories, 0 g protein, 2 g carbohydrates, 4 g fat (0.6 g saturated), 0 mg cholesterol, 0 g fiber, 154 mg sodium

Almond Dressing

MAKES ½ CUP DRESSING

I made this dressing when I was experimenting with a diet that included lots of raw veggies, and I love the taste that the sweet, crunchy almond butter lends it. This dressing is a great option for people who suffer from celiac disease or who have allergies to peanuts but not almonds.

¼ cup unsalted almond butter

2 tablespoons sherry or apple cider vinegar

1 tablespoon reduced-sodium soy sauce

1 small shallot, quartered

Place the almond butter, vinegar, soy sauce, and shallots in a minichopper or blender. Process until smooth. Serve immediately or refrigerate for up to 2 weeks.

Per serving (2 tablespoons): 108 calories, 3 g protein, 5 g carbohydrates, 9.5 g fat (1 g saturated), 0 mg cholesterol, 1 g fiber, 146 mg sodium

Green Beans with Almonds and Lemon Pepper Croutons

SERVES 4

I love the flavor combo of lemon and pepper—it gives a tangy zest to veggies. In this dish, the lemon pepper croutons lend a delicious crunch.

  1 pound green beans, trimmed and cut into thirds
  1 tablespoon olive oil
  1 small whole wheat bun (about 2 ounces), cubed
  2 tablespoons slivered almonds
  1 teaspoon freshly grated lemon zest
  ½ teaspoon coarsely ground black pepper
  ¼ teaspoon paprika
  2 tablespoons grated Parmesan cheese
  ¼ teaspoon salt

In a large saucepan, bring 1 inch of water to a boil. Add the green beans and cover. Cook 4 to 5 minutes, until the green beans are tender crisp. Set aside.

Heat the oil in a large skillet over medium heat. Add the bread and almonds, then sprinkle in the lemon zest, pepper, and paprika. Toss the bread with tongs and cook 2 to 3 minutes, until the bread starts to brown. Add the green beans, Parmesan, and salt. Toss well to coat and serve immediately.

Per serving (1¼ cups): 166 calories, 7 g protein, 21 g carbohydrates, 7 g fat (1.4 g saturated), 2 mg cholesterol, 6 g fiber, 309 mg sodium

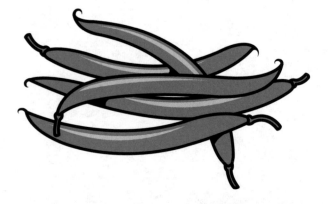

Honey-Roasted Baby Carrots with Raisins

SERVES 4

Simple and sweet, roasted carrots are a fast and easy side dish that goes well with almost any meal, including your holiday favorites like roasted leg of lamb or stuffed turkey.

2 pounds baby carrots
2 tablespoons butter
2 tablespoons honey
2 tablespoons brown sugar
¼ cup raisins
1 teaspoon ground cinnamon
¼ teaspoon ground cloves
1 orange, zested and juiced

Preheat the oven to 350°F. In a large stockpot, bring 1 inch of water to a boil. Add the carrots. Steam 7 to 8 minutes, checking the water level halfway through cooking and adding ¼ cup of water if needed. Transfer the carrots to a 7 x 12-inch pan along with the butter, honey, brown sugar, raisins, cinnamon, cloves, orange zest, and orange juice. Stir well to combine. Bake 15 to 20 minutes, until the carrots start to lightly brown. Serve immediately.

Per serving (1 cup): 231 calories, 2 g protein, 45 g carbohydrates, 6 g fat (3.7 g saturated), 15 mg cholesterol, 8 g fiber, 222 mg sodium

Simple Sautéed Spinach with Garlic and Chile Flakes

SERVES 4

Spinach is one of the most nutritious vegetables, and I love this fresh, fast way to eat it. This preparation tastes mild, will appeal even to those who don't love spinach, and can go along with almost any main course.

4 teaspoons olive oil

1 garlic clove, cut in half

¼ teaspoon red chile pepper flakes

2 10-ounce bags baby or prewashed spinach

½ teaspoon salt

Heat half the oil in a large skillet over high heat. Add the garlic and cook about 1 minute, until the garlic lightly browns. Add the pepper flakes and half the spinach, then sprinkle with half the salt. Press the spinach down with a pot lid. Add 2 tablespoons of water and turn the spinach with tongs. Cook 3 to 4 minutes, turning the spinach often, until it is wilted. Transfer the wilted spinach to a large bowl or plate. Repeat the cooking process with the remaining oil, spinach, and salt. Stir the two batches together and serve immediately.

Per serving (½ cup): 100 calories, 3 g protein, 15 g carbohydrates, 4.5 g fat (0.6 g saturated), 0 mg cholesterol, 7 g fiber, 516 mg sodium

Skinny Secret

Spinach is not only the superhero of the veggie world but it's a favorite of home cooks since it cooks really fast.

Stir-Fried Garlic Broccoli

SERVES 4

Chinese takeout is so good because it's fast and flavorful and usually has a thick, rich-tasting sauce. This recipe has all of those features without the grease and with the goodness of broccoli, which boasts lots of vitamin C and calcium.

- ¾ cup reduced-sodium, fat-free beef broth
- 2 teaspoons cornstarch
- 2 garlic cloves, minced
- 2 teaspoons grated fresh ginger
- 1 tablespoon reduced-sodium soy sauce
- 1 tablespoon dry sherry (optional)
- 1 teaspoon brown sugar
- 1 tablespoon sesame oil
- 1 head broccoli, cut into florets, stem peeled and chopped
  Juice of 2 limes

Place the broth, cornstarch, garlic, ginger, soy sauce, sherry if using, and brown sugar in a medium bowl. Whisk until smooth.

Heat a large skillet or wok over high heat. Add the oil and broccoli. Cook 4 to 6 minutes, until the broccoli starts to brown. Reduce the heat to low. Add the sauce and cook 1 to 2 minutes longer, until a thick sauce forms. Add the lime juice and stir well. Serve immediately.

Per serving (1 cup): 111 calories, 6 g protein, 16 g carbohydrates, 4 g fat (0.6 g saturated), 0 mg cholesterol, 5 g fiber, 285 mg sodium

Warm Creamed Spinach Minus the Heavy Cream

SERVES 4

I've always loved ordering creamed spinach in restaurants because it's savory, soft, and scented with spices. This version retains its bright green color, and still has a creamy texture without the heavy cream.

- 1 tablespoon olive oil
- 1 small onion, chopped
- 2 cloves garlic, chopped
- 1 tablespoon whole wheat flour
- 1/4 teaspoon freshly grated nutmeg
- 1 cup fat-free milk
- 2 pounds baby spinach
- 1/4 cup plain, fat-free Greek yogurt
- 1/4 cup grated Parmesan cheese

Skinny Secret

If I were on a desert island and could eat only one vegetable, I would pick spinach, the super-hero of the vegetable world. Fast cooking, fresh spinach tastes awesome and provides high levels of vitamins like A, B_2, B_6, C, and K plus minerals like calcium, iron, manganese, and potassium!

Heat the oil in a large stockpot over medium heat. Cook the onions and garlic 8 to 10 minutes, stirring occasionally. Add a tablespoon of water if the onions stick. Add the flour and nutmeg. Cook 1 to 2 minutes, mashing the flour into the onions with a wooden spoon. Add the milk and whisk. Bring to a slow boil, whisking until a thick sauce starts to form. Add the spinach and stir with tongs to coat. Cover and cook 2 to 3 minutes, until the spinach wilts. Remove the pot from the heat and stir in the yogurt and Parmesan. Serve immediately.

Per serving (3/4 cup): 169 calories, 9 g protein, 28 g carbohydrates, 5 g fat (1.4 g saturated), 4 mg cholesterol, 11 g fiber, 443 mg sodium

Buttermilk Biscuits

MAKES 12 BISCUITS

If you're not serving these buttermilk biscuits the same day you make them, place them in a large zipper-lock bag and store in the freezer. They warm up perfectly in a toaster oven for a fast breakfast bite.

3½ cups whole wheat pastry flour or white whole wheat flour, plus ¼ cup for rolling

2 teaspoons baking powder

½ teaspoon baking soda

¼ teaspoon salt

¼ teaspoon paprika

10 tablespoons trans-fat-free margarine, cut into 1-inch pieces

1 cup low-fat (1 percent) buttermilk

Preheat the oven to 400°F. Place the flour, baking powder, baking soda, salt, and paprika in a food processor and pulse to combine. Add the margarine. Pulse 8 to 10 times, until pea-size crumbs start to form. Add the buttermilk and pulse 4 or 5 times, until a uniform smooth dough forms.

Preheat the oven to 400°F. Turn out the dough onto a countertop sprinkled with the remaining flour. Roll the dough into a 2-inch-thick sheet. Dip a small juice glass or 3-inch biscuit cutter into flour and cut out rounds of biscuits. Transfer the biscuits to a cookie sheet. Bring the remaining dough together and cut out additional biscuits; you should have 12 total. Bake 8 to 10 minutes, until the biscuits are cooked through. Cool completely on a wire rack, then store the biscuits in an airtight container on the countertop for up to 3 days.

Per serving (1 biscuit): 208 calories, 4 g protein, 27 g carbohydrates, 8.6 g fat (2.4 g saturated), 1 mg cholesterol, 3.5 g fiber, 265 mg sodium

Whole Wheat Garlic Bread

SERVES 8

Homemade bread is so flavorful, and you definitely won't miss all the preservatives that you find in a lot of commercial loaves. You can skip the garlic spread and just enjoy this recipe as a plain whole wheat baguette.

2½ cups white whole wheat flour, plus ¼ cup for rolling

⅓ cup carrot juice

2 tablespoons ground flaxseed

1 1¼-ounce packet dry yeast

1 teaspoon granulated sugar

½ teaspoon salt

1 cup warm water

Nonstick cooking spray

GARLIC SPREAD

¼ cup fresh flat-leaf parsley, chopped

2 garlic cloves, minced

2 tablespoons trans-fat-free margarine

1 tablespoon reduced-fat cream cheese

¼ teaspoon salt

Place the flour, carrot juice, flaxseed, yeast, sugar, and salt in a food processor. Pulse to mix. With the motor running, pour in the warm water. A soft dough should start to form and begin to stick to the blade. Let the dough ride the blade 1 to 2 minutes, until the dough is smooth and bounces back when you squeeze it. Coat a large bowl with cooking spray. Place the dough inside and cover tightly with plastic wrap. Let the dough rise 1 to 2 hours, until it doubles in size.

In a small bowl, combine the parsley, garlic, margarine, cream cheese, and salt. Mash with the back of a spoon until smooth. Refrigerate until ready to use.

Preheat the oven to 350°F. Punch the dough down and turn it out onto the counter-top. Sprinkle the dough with the remaining flour. Roll the dough into a 12-inch-long by 2-inch-wide log. Transfer the dough to an ungreased baking sheet. Bake 20 to 25 minutes, until the dough is crusty on the outside and cooked in the center. Cool on a wire rack 15 to 20 minutes. Cut the warm bread in half lengthwise and smear with the garlic spread. Cut into 8 pieces and serve immediately.

Per serving (1 piece): 167 calories, 6 g protein, 29 g carbohydrates, 3.6 g fat (1 g saturated), 1 mg cholesterol, 4 g fiber, 111 mg sodium

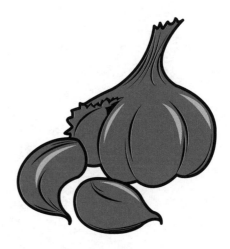

Desserts

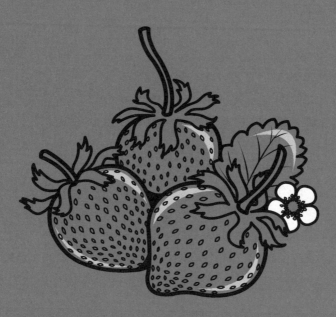

131 CRUSTLESS APPLE PIE

132 BANANA CREAM PIE

134 BLUEBERRY COBBLER WITH YOGURT TOPPING

136 CARROT CAKE WITH APPLESAUCE AND CARROT JUICE

138 CHOCOLATE ANGEL FOOD CUPCAKES WITH ANGELIC ICING

140 MY GRANNY'S CINNAMON COFFEE CAKE THE SKINNY WAY

142 SINFUL CHOCOLATE CAKE MADE WITH RAISINS
AND BITTERSWEET MORSELS

143 ITALIAN CHEESECAKE

144 TIRAMISU PARFAITS

146 SLENDER BLONDIE BROWNIES WITH WALNUTS, CHOCOLATE CHIPS,
AND PRUNES

148 APPLE STRUDEL WITH WALNUT CRUMBLE TOPPING

150 BANANA BREAD

152 ZUCCHINI BREAD FIT FOR BREAKFAST, TOO

154 RICOTTA STRAWBERRY SHORTCAKE PARFAITS

155 CHOCOLATE-COVERED PRETZELS AND FRUIT

156 FROZEN FRUIT SKEWERS

157 CHOCOLATE PUDDING POPS

158 CHERRY SHERBET

159 FROZEN COCONUT YOGURT

160 VANILLA BEAN "ICE CREAM"

161 HOT FUDGE SUNDAES WITH VANILLA BEAN FROZEN YOGURT

Crustless Apple Pie

SERVES 8

Apple pie crusts are loaded with butter, and a store-bought pie can contain lots of harmful preservatives and trans fats. This version has a topping instead of a crust and is made with simple, fresh ingredients.

       2 cups pancake mix, such as Bisquick
       1 cup rolled oats
       1 teaspoon pumpkin pie spice
      ¼ teaspoon ground cloves
      ½ cup plus 1 tablespoon trans-fat-free margarine
      ½ cup fat-free milk
       4 apples (about 2 pounds), such as Gala or Golden Delicious, cored, peeled, and sliced
       1 cup brown sugar
       2 tablespoons apple cider vinegar
          Juice of 1 lemon (about ¼ cup)
          Nonstick cooking spray

Preheat the oven to 400°F. In a large bowl, place the pancake mix, rolled oats, pumpkin pie spice, and ground cloves. Mix well with a wooden spoon. Add the ½ cup margarine. With your fingertips, rub the margarine into the flour mixture until pea-size crumbs form. Add the milk and stir 3 or 4 times, until a dough forms.

Heat a large ovenproof skillet over high heat. Add 1 tablespoon of margarine and the apple slices. Reduce the heat to medium and cook 4 to 5 minutes, stirring occasionally, until the apples start to brown. Add a tablespoon of water if they stick. Add the sugar, vinegar, and lemon juice. Cook 4 to 5 minutes, until the apples are soft.

Spoon the topping over the apples. Coat the top with a light layer of cooking spray. Bake 9 to 10 minutes, until the topping is cooked through. Spoon into small bowls and serve immediately.

Per serving (½ cup): 412 calories, 5 g protein, 66 g carbohydrates, 15.8 g fat (4.3 g saturated), 0 mg cholesterol, 3 g fiber, 496 mg sodium

Banana Cream Pie

SERVES 8

Old-fashioned desserts can be pretty and festive. This pie is made with a lot less sugar than the traditional version and has heart-healthy flaxseed added to the rich pudding filling.

GRAHAM CRUST

1½ cups whole wheat graham crackers (about 8 grahams)

  2 tablespoons trans-fat-free margarine, melted

FILLING

½ cup whole wheat flour

⅓ cup granulated sugar

½ teaspoon ground cinnamon

2 tablespoons ground flaxseed

¼ teaspoon salt

2½ cups fat-free milk

3 egg yolks, lightly beaten

2 teaspoons vanilla extract

1 tablespoon trans-fat-free margarine

3 ripe bananas, thinly sliced (about 1 pound)

MERINGUE

4 egg whites

¼ teaspoon cream of tartar

⅓ cup granulated sugar

Preheat the oven to 375°F. Place the graham crackers in a food processor and pulse them into fine crumbs. Drizzle in the melted margarine and pulse again. Spoon the mixture into the bottom of an 8-inch pie plate and press with your fingers to form an even crust. Bake 8 to 10 minutes until crust is firm. Transfer to a wire rack to cool.

Whisk the flour, sugar, cinnamon, flaxseed, and salt in a large saucepan off the heat. Add the milk gradually, stirring until smooth. Cook the mixture over medium-high heat, until it boils, stirring constantly. Transfer 1 cup of the liquid into a mug. Whisk in the egg yolks. Slowly mix the contents of the mug back into the liquid in the saucepan. Remove from the heat and stir in the vanilla and margarine. Cool 10 to 15 minutes.

Place the bananas on top of the graham crust, pour in the filling, and smooth with a rubber spatula.

In a large bowl, beat the egg whites and cream of tartar until frothy with an electric mixer set on high speed. Add the sugar gradually. Continue beating the egg whites, until they hold a glossy peak.

Spoon the meringue onto the filling, spreading the egg whites to the edge of the crust with the back of a spoon. To make decorative peaks for the top of the pie, touch the back of the spoon to the egg whites and lift up. Bake 10 to 15 minutes or until the meringue is nicely browned. Transfer to a wire rack to cool completely. Serve at room temperature or chill uncovered for 1 hour before slicing.

Per serving (1 slice): 273 calories, 9 g protein, 44 g carbohydrates, 7.4 g fat (1.7 g saturated), 80 mg cholesterol, 3 g fiber, 260 mg sodium

Blueberry Cobbler with Yogurt Topping

SERVES 8

Not too sweet, not too tart, berry cobbler is the perfect ending to a summer barbecue or Indian summer meal. My husband thinks the orange zest makes this recipe, but I like the zing that ground cardamom adds to the topping.

- 1 cup fat-free Greek yogurt
- 2 tablespoons confectioners' sugar
- 2 pints fresh blueberries
- 2 teaspoons orange zest
- 2 tablespoons light brown sugar
- 2 tablespoons ground flaxseed
- 1 tablespoon whole wheat pastry flour

TOPPING

- ½ cup old-fashioned oats
- ½ cup whole wheat pastry flour
- ½ cup packed light brown sugar
- 1 teaspoon baking powder
- ½ teaspoon ground cinnamon
- ½ teaspoon ground cardamom
- ¼ teaspoon salt
- ⅓ cup trans-fat-free margarine, chilled
- 2 teaspoons ice water

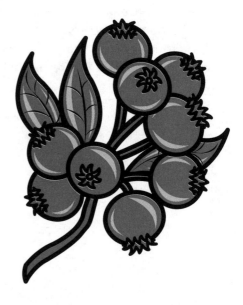

Preheat the oven to 375°F. In a medium bowl, mix the yogurt with the confectioners' sugar. Refrigerate until ready to use. Place the blueberries, orange zest, brown sugar, flaxseed, and flour in a large bowl. Mix well to combine. Transfer to an 8 x 8-inch ungreased baking dish.

Place the oats in a food processor and pulse until a chunky flour forms. Add the flour, brown sugar, baking powder, cinnamon, cardamom, and salt to the food processor bowl and pulse 2 or 3 times to combine. Add the margarine and ice water, then pulse 7 or 8 times, until pea-size crumbs start to form. Do not overmix.

Sprinkle the topping over the fruit and bake 35 to 40 minutes, until the berries are hot and the topping is cooked through. Cool 5 minutes. Spoon the yogurt mixture over top and serve.

Per serving (½ cup): 249 calories, 5 g protein, 41 g carbohydrates, 7.7 g fat (1.8 g saturated), 0 mg cholesterol, 4 g fiber, 199 mg sodium

Skinny Secret

Kids think ground flaxseed looks like cookie crumbs or ground sesame seeds. It's the perfect nutritional supplement to add to desserts without having to hear, "Yuck, what is that?"

Carrot Cake with Applesauce and Carrot Juice

SERVES 10

Carrot cake is one of those desserts that seems healthy because it contains carrots. But it actually can be very heavy, since it's typically packed with oil and heavy icing. The ingredient list for this light recipe is lengthy, but it's well worth it! It also comes together quickly when you use an electric mixer.

Nonstick cooking spray

2 cups whole wheat flour

2 teaspoons ground cinnamon

1 teaspoon baking soda

1 teaspoon baking powder

½ teaspoon ground allspice

¼ teaspoon salt

4 egg whites

¾ cup firmly packed brown sugar

½ cup low-fat (1 percent) buttermilk

½ cup unsweetened applesauce

½ cup carrot juice

¼ cup vegetable oil

¼ cup granulated sugar

3 cups lightly packed, shredded peeled carrots

½ cup prunes, cut into small pieces

CREAM CHEESE FROSTING

1 8-ounce package fat-free cream cheese, at room temperature

6 tablespoons trans-fat-free margarine, at room temperature

¼ cup confectioners' sugar

1 teaspoon vanilla extract

Preheat the oven to 350°F. Coat two 9-inch cake pans with the cooking spray. On a piece of waxed paper, sift together the flour, cinnamon, baking soda, baking powder, allspice, and salt. Using an electric mixer set on medium speed, beat the egg whites, brown sugar, buttermilk, applesauce, carrot juice, oil, and granulated sugar in a large bowl until well blended. Add the flour mixture and carrots and prunes all at one time and mix on low until the flour is just combined.

Divide the batter evenly between the prepared pans. Bake until a toothpick inserted into the centers comes out clean, 35 to 40 minutes. Transfer to racks and let cool in the pans for 15 minutes. Invert the cakes onto the racks and let cool completely.

Meanwhile, put the cream cheese and margarine in a large bowl. Using an electric mixer set on medium-high speed, beat until smooth. Reduce the speed to low, add the confectioners' sugar, and beat until smooth. Beat in the vanilla until well blended.

Place one cake layer on a plate. Spread 1½ cups of the frosting over the top. Place the second cake layer on top. Spread the remaining frosting decoratively over the top and sides of the cake. Serve immediately or cover with a cake dome and refrigerate for up to 2 days.

Per serving (1 slice): 355 calories, 9 g protein, 55 g carbohydrates, 12 g fat (3 g saturated), 2 mg cholesterol, 5 g fiber, 474 mg sodium

Skinny Secret

Fruit is Mother Nature's dessert and is an excellent base for homemade treats. When you want to replace some of the oil called for in traditional recipes, don't limit yourself to the "applesauce trick"—pureed canned pears, peaches, apricots in natural juice, and fresh bananas can also be used as oil substitutes.

Chocolate Angel Food Cupcakes with Angelic Icing

MAKES 12 CUPCAKES

I was never a fan of angel food cake or so-called diet cakes growing up, but this chocolate version has an alluring texture. I call the icing "angelic" because it's a sweet, pink icing that is light and low in sugar compared to icing on the calorie killers that are store-bought cupcakes.

½ cup fat-free milk
1 tablespoon balsamic vinegar
1 teaspoon vanilla extract
¼ cup trans-fat-free margarine
½ cup granulated sugar
2 ripe bananas, mashed (about ¾ cup)
2 egg whites
3 tablespoons unsweetened cocoa powder
½ teaspoon baking soda
½ teaspoon salt
1 cup whole wheat pastry flour

ANGELIC ICING

1 tablespoon reduced-fat cream cheese
1 tablespoon confectioners' sugar
1 tablespoon whole wheat pastry flour
½ ripe banana

Preheat the oven to 350°F. Line a 12-cup muffin tin with paper liners.

Place the milk, vinegar, and vanilla in a small bowl. Stir to mix and set aside. Place the margarine and sugar in a large bowl. Using an electric mixer set on high speed, beat until well combined. Add the mashed bananas and egg whites. Beat on medium speed until well combined. Sprinkle in the cocoa, baking soda, and salt. Mix on low speed. Alternating the milk mixture with the flour, add to the banana mixture in two additions, mixing on low speed until just combined.

Fill each paper liner three-fourths full with batter. Bake 30 to 35 minutes, until the cupcakes puff and spring back when touched. Transfer the cupcakes to a wire rack to cool completely.

Meanwhile, place the cream cheese, confectioners' sugar, and flour in a large bowl and beat with the electric mixer until smooth. Add the banana piece and mix well on high speed. Drizzle the banana icing onto the cupcakes and serve immediately or cover and refrigerate for up to 2 days.

Per serving (1 cupcake): 142 calories, 3 g protein, 24 g carbohydrates, 4.2 g fat (1 g saturated), 1 mg cholesterol, 2 g fiber, 204 mg sodium

My Granny's Cinnamon Coffee Cake the Skinny Way

SERVES 8

One of my favorite breakfasts as a little girl was a small slice of cake. With this coffee cake I can still have my cake for breakfast once in a while without worrying about loading up on fat and sugar.

Nonstick cooking spray
½ cup packed brown sugar
½ cup chopped walnuts
1 teaspoon ground cinnamon
1¼ cups cake flour
1¼ cups white whole wheat flour or whole wheat pastry flour
2 teaspoons baking powder
½ teaspoon baking soda
¼ teaspoon salt
1 cup low-fat (1 percent) buttermilk
1 8-ounce can pears packed in water, drained
¼ cup trans-fat-free margarine
½ cup granulated sugar
3 egg whites
2 teaspoons vanilla extract

Preheat the oven to 350°F. Coat an 8-inch round springform pan with cooking spray. On a sheet of waxed paper, mix the brown sugar, walnuts, and cinnamon with your fingertips.

Place the cake flour, wheat flour, baking powder, baking soda, and salt in a large bowl. Stir until combined. Place the buttermilk and pears in a blender; process until smooth.

In another large bowl, beat the margarine and granulated sugar with an electric mixer set on high speed until well combined. Add the egg whites and vanilla; mix well. Add the flour mixture, alternating with the buttermilk-pear mixture, in three additions.

Spoon the batter into the pan. Sprinkle the walnut-cinnamon mixture evenly over the batter. With a knife, swirl the walnut mixture into the batter. Bake 55 to 60 minutes, until a toothpick comes out clean when inserted. Transfer the pan to a wire rack and cool 10 minutes. Run a knife around the inside of the pan. Remove the cake from the springform and cool completely.

Per serving (1 slice): 360 calories, 8 g protein, 61 g carbohydrates, 10 g fat (2 g saturated), 2 mg cholesterol, 3 g fiber, 356 mg sodium

Sinful Chocolate Cake Made with Raisins and Bittersweet Morsels

SERVES 12

I like a moist, dense, yet soft cake. This cake is so rich it doesn't need icing, and the raisins add a bit of chewy sweetness. It's like a devil's food cake without all the devilish fat from the two sticks of butter used in the traditional version.

      Nonstick cooking spray
½   cup unsweetened cocoa powder
½   cup raisins
 1   cup boiling water
½   cup fat-free sour cream
 1   teaspoon baking powder
⅔   cup packed light brown sugar
½   cup bittersweet chocolate morsels
¼   cup canola or vegetable oil
 2   large egg whites
 1   tablespoon vanilla extract
 1   teaspoon baking soda
¼   teaspoon salt
 1   cup whole wheat pastry flour

Preheat the oven to 350°F. Coat a 9 x 12-inch casserole dish with cooking spray. Place the cocoa and raisins in a small bowl with the boiling water. Set aside.

Place the sour cream and baking powder in a coffee mug. Stir and set aside. Place the brown sugar, chocolate morsels, oil, egg whites, and vanilla in a large bowl. Using an electric mixer, beat on high speed until smooth. Add the cocoa raisin mixture. Sprinkle the baking soda and salt over the sugar mixture. Add the flour, alternating with the sour cream mixture in two additions. Transfer the batter to the casserole dish and bake 20 to 25 minutes, until the center of the cake springs back to the touch or a toothpick comes out clean when inserted in the center.

Per serving (1 slice): 198 calories, 3 g protein, 33 g carbohydrates, 7.3 g fat (2 g saturated), 1 mg cholesterol, 2 g fiber, 210 mg sodium

Italian Cheesecake

SERVES 8

This is the "angel food" version of cheesecake; it's much lighter than traditional cheesecake. Eating lighter desserts has its benefits, since rich desserts can be rough not only on the waistline but also on the digestion at the end of the night.

Nonstick cooking spray
8 egg whites
¼ teaspoon salt
½ pound fat-free ricotta cheese (heaping ¾ cup)
½ pound part-skim ricotta cheese (heaping ¾ cup)
½ cup granulated sugar
⅓ cup whole wheat flour
¼ teaspoon ground cinnamon
2 teaspoons vanilla extract
1 small orange, zested and juiced
1 pint strawberries, stemmed and thinly sliced
2 tablespoons fresh mint, thinly sliced

Preheat the oven to 300°F. Set the rack in the middle of the oven. Coat a 9½-inch springform pan with cooking spray. Place the egg whites and salt in a large bowl. Using an electric mixer set on high speed, beat 3 to 4 minutes, until soft peaks start to form. Set aside. Place both types of ricotta in another large mixing bowl; beat with an electric mixer until combined. Reduce the speed to low and beat in the sugar, flour, cinnamon, vanilla, and orange zest.

Using a rubber spatula, fold the ricotta mixture into the egg whites in three additions, stirring gently so that you do not deflate the egg whites. Pour the mixture into the prepared pan and smooth the top. Bake 50 to 60 minutes, until the top is lightly browned and the cake jiggles slightly. Cool the cheesecake on a wire rack.

Stir the orange juice, strawberries, and mint in a small bowl. Run a knife around the inside of the pan to loosen the cake. Remove the ring and chill the cake covered at least 1 hour. Cut into eight pieces and top with strawberries.

Per serving (1 slice): 161 calories, 11 g protein, 24 g carbohydrates, 2.5 g fat (1.4 g saturated), 11 mg cholesterol, 1.6 g fiber, 200 mg sodium

Tiramisu Parfaits

SERVES 4

I like my morning coffee strong, but sometimes there's a cup at the bottom of the pot that I can't finish. I store it in the fridge and use it to make this simple but elegant dessert.

CHOCOLATE FILLING

- 2 cups fat-free milk
- 2 tablespoons unsweetened cocoa powder
- 1/4 cup confectioners' sugar
- 2 tablespoons cornstarch

CREAMY FILLING

- 1 cup unsweetened applesauce
- 1 cup low-fat (1 percent) cottage cheese
- 1/4 cup reduced-fat cream cheese
- 2 tablespoons confectioners' sugar
- 1 teaspoon vanilla extract

PARFAITS

- 8 large low-fat store-bought biscotti
- 2 tablespoons confectioners' sugar
- 1 cup strongly brewed coffee, cooled to room temperature
- 4 teaspoons unsweetened cocoa powder

Place the milk, cocoa powder, sugar, and cornstarch in a medium saucepan. Place over medium heat and cook 4 to 5 minutes, whisking often, until a thick sauce forms.

Place the applesauce, cottage cheese, cream cheese, sugar, and vanilla in a mini-chopper. Process until smooth.

Break the biscotti in half. Place a piece of biscotti in the bottoms of each of four parfait glasses. Mix the confectioners' sugar with the coffee, then spoon 1 table-spoon of the coffee mixture into each glass. Dot each with the chocolate filling and then the creamy filling. Repeat the layers three times, ending with the creamy filling. Sprinkle each parfait with 1 teaspoon cocoa powder. Cover and refrigerate at least 1 hour before serving.

Per serving (about 1 cup): 349 calories, 17 g protein, 60 g carbohydrates, 6.5 g fat (2.2 g saturated), 11 mg cholesterol, 5 g fiber, 418 mg sodium

Slender Blondie Brownies with Walnuts, Chocolate Chips, and Prunes

MAKES 12 BROWNIES

When I was a kid, I was a major sneak-eater. I'd stuff the empty wrappers from prepackaged brownies under the sofa. Now, if I really want a brownie, I don't need to sneak it; I have the healthier version in plain sight.

Nonstick cooking spray
3/4 cup white whole wheat flour
1/2 teaspoon baking powder
1/4 teaspoon baking soda
1/8 teaspoon salt
1/4 cup canola oil
2/3 cup packed light or dark brown sugar
2 egg whites
1 tablespoon vanilla extract
1/2 cup chopped prunes
1/4 cup chopped walnuts
1/4 cup bittersweet chocolate morsels

Skinny Secret

"White" whole wheat flour is a lot softer than regular stone ground whole wheat flour and makes for tender baked goods.

Preheat the oven to 350°F. Coat a 9-inch square pan with cooking spray. Sift the flour, baking powder, baking soda, and salt onto a piece of waxed paper or aluminum foil. Set aside.

In a large bowl, beat the oil and sugar until smooth, 1 to 2 minutes. Mix in the egg whites and vanilla. With a wooden spoon, stir in the flour mixture until just combined. Fold in the prunes, walnuts, and morsels.

Spread the batter in the pan. Bake 25 to 30 minutes or until a wooden pick inserted in the center comes out clean or with moist-looking crumbs. Cool 5 minutes in the pan, then turn out onto a wire rack to cool completely. Cut into 12 pieces and store in an airtight container for up to 5 days.

Per serving (1 piece): 169 calories, 2 g protein, 25 g carbohydrates, 7.2 g fat (1 g saturated), 0 mg cholesterol, 1 g fiber, 81 mg sodium

Apple Strudel with Walnut Crumble Topping

SERVES 8

I used to gobble up those toaster strudel-like treats filled with artificial fruit flavors. This version is just as delicious, but it doesn't contain any unrecognizable ingredients! The topping adds crunch that contrasts with the soft filling made with real fruit.

TOPPING

¼   cup walnuts

2   tablespoons oats

2   tablespoons brown sugar

1   teaspoon ground cinnamon

¼   teaspoon salt

STRUDEL

Nonstick cooking spray

3   large apples, such as Golden Delicious or Gala, peeled, cored, and thinly sliced

½   cup raisins

¼   cup prunes, chopped

1   small orange, zested and juiced

2   tablespoons brown sugar

2   tablespoons whole wheat flour

1   teaspoon ground cinnamon

¼   cup water

1   tablespoon butter

12   sheets frozen phyllo dough, defrosted

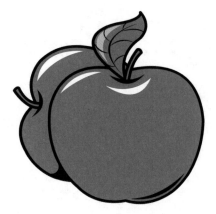

Combine the walnuts, oats, brown sugar, cinnamon, and salt in a small bowl. Mix together with your fingertips or a spoon until well combined.

Preheat the oven to 350°F. Coat an 8 x 12-inch baking dish with cooking spray. In a large saucepan, combine the apple slices, raisins, prunes, orange zest, orange juice, brown sugar, flour, cinnamon, and water. Stir well. Over medium-low heat, bring to a slow simmer. Cook 10 to 15 minutes, until a thick sauce forms and the apples are tender. Stir in the butter and set aside to cool for 5 minutes.

Lay half the phyllo sheets across the baking dish so that the edges of the dough hang over the sides. Pour in half of the apple mixture. Top with the other half of the phyllo sheets. Spoon in the remaining apple filling. Fold the two longer sides of the dough on top of each other as if folding a shirt and tuck the shorter ends underneath. Sprinkle the top with the walnut mixture. Coat with a thin layer of cooking spray and bake 15 to 20 minutes, until the phyllo is crisp.

Per serving (1 piece): 255 calories, 4 g protein, 50 g carbohydrates, 5.5 g fat (1 g saturated), 0 mg cholesterol, 4 g fiber, 225 mg sodium

Skinny Secret

Cherishing fresh, seasonal ingredients is a smart move. Fresh ingredients are often tastier and usually cheaper, and purchasing locally grown food is good for the environment too.

Banana Bread

SERVES 14

Whole wheat baked goods sometimes get a bad rap. Even though this bread is made with 100 percent whole wheat, it's still moist and tender. The brown sugar swirl on top adds a hint of sweet crunch without being overwhelmingly sugary.

    Nonstick cooking spray
1½ cups mashed bananas (about 3 bananas or 1 pound)
⅔ cup packed brown sugar
½ cup low-fat (1 percent) buttermilk
2 egg whites
¼ cup canola or vegetable oil
1 tablespoon balsamic vinegar
1 tablespoon vanilla extract
1 teaspoon baking soda
¼ teaspoon baking powder
1⅔ cups white whole wheat flour or whole wheat pastry flour

SWIRL

½ cup chopped walnuts
2 tablespoons brown sugar
2 teaspoons ground cinnamon

Skinny Secret

I add a little vinegar to some of my baked goods to tenderize the whole grain flour. I especially like balsamic vinegar, since it has a chocolaty color.

Preheat the oven to 325°F. Coat a 1-pound loaf pan with cooking spray. Place the mashed bananas in a large bowl. Add the brown sugar, buttermilk, egg whites, oil, vinegar, vanilla, baking soda, and baking powder. Using an electric mixer, beat 1 to 2 minutes, until the banana is well combined with the other ingredients. Sprinkle the flour over the banana mixture. Using a wooden spoon, mix until the flour is just incorporated—there will be dry spots. Transfer the batter to the loaf pan.

Sprinkle the walnuts, brown sugar, and cinnamon over the top. With the tip of the knife, swirl the topping into the batter, making 7 or 8 turns. Bake 45 to 50 minutes, until a toothpick comes out clean when inserted in the center. Cool 5 minutes before removing the bread from the pan. Cool completely on a wire rack, then store in an airtight container for up to 3 days.

Per serving (1 slice): 189 calories, 4 g protein, 30 g carbohydrates, 7 g fat (0.5 g saturated), 4 mg cholesterol, 2 g fiber, 119 mg sodium

Zucchini Bread Fit for Breakfast, Too

SERVES 12

I call this Fit for Breakfast since it is a low-sugar baked good that could serve as a whole grain morning treat. If you want to have it for dessert, just top it with a little confectioners' sugar and some fresh berries.

- Nonstick cooking spray
- 2 cups whole wheat pastry flour
- 1 cup cooked quinoa
- 2 teaspoons baking powder
- 1 teaspoon baking soda
- 2 teaspoons ground cinnamon
- ¼ teaspoon ground cloves
- ¼ teaspoon freshly ground nutmeg
- ¼ teaspoon salt
- ¾ cup granulated sugar
- 2 eggs
- 2 egg whites
- ¼ cup canola oil
- 1 teaspoon vanilla extract
- 2 cups shredded zucchini (from 1 medium zucchini, about ½ pound)
- ½ cup chopped pineapple
- ¼ cup golden raisins

Skinny Secret

Add leftover cooked grains to baked goods. You can even stir them into waffle or pancake batter for extra whole grain goodness.

Preheat the oven to 350°F. Coat a Bundt cake pan with cooking spray, then coat the pan with flour and set aside. In a large bowl, combine the flour, quinoa, baking powder, baking soda, cinnamon, cloves, nutmeg, and salt.

In another large bowl, mix the sugar, eggs, egg whites, oil, and vanilla with a wooden spoon until smooth. Stir in the flour mixture until almost combined; the mixture will still have dry spots. Add the zucchini, pineapple, and raisins. Transfer the batter to the Bundt pan and bake 60 to 75 minutes, until a knife comes out clean.

Per serving (1 slice): 216 calories, 5 g protein, 35 g carbohydrates, 6 g fat (0.6 g saturated), 35 mg cholesterol, 3 g fiber, 245 mg sodium

Ricotta Strawberry Shortcake Parfaits

SERVES 4

I love desserts that look decadent but are actually light on sugar and packed with fruit so you can feast your eyes even as you make a better choice for your body. This gorgeous parfait is fit for an elegant dinner party or a special after-dinner surprise for kids.

1 pint strawberries, thinly sliced

1 tablespoon balsamic vinegar

1 tablespoon confectioners' sugar

2 tablespoons fresh mint leaves, plus 4 sprigs for garnish

1 small orange, zested and juiced

1 cup part-skim ricotta cheese

1 tablespoon honey

4 sponge cake shells

Place the strawberries, vinegar, sugar, 2 tablespoons mint, orange zest, and orange juice in a medium bowl; toss to coat. In another bowl, mix the ricotta and honey.

Cut each sponge cake shell in half horizontally. Press one half into the bottoms of each of four glasses. Spoon strawberries over the cake and add a little of the juice. Then spoon on 2 tablespoons of the ricotta mixture. Repeat with another layer of sponge cake and strawberries, ending with the ricotta. Garnish with the mint sprigs. Cover and chill at least 1 hour or until the topping is firm.

Per serving (1 cup): 261 calories, 10 g protein, 43 g carbohydrates, 6.2 g fat (3.3 g saturated), 58 mg cholesterol, 3 g fiber, 173 mg sodium

Chocolate-Covered Pretzels and Fruit

SERVES 12

When I was a little girl, my granny used to dress me up and take me to Kaufmann's, a fancy department store that had a gourmet chocolate counter. I'd always pick out the salty-sweet chocolate-covered pretzel as my treat. My version is still a treat, yet lighter in the fat department.

    4 large whole wheat pretzel sticks
    1 orange, peeled and sectioned
    4 large strawberries
    2 ounces bittersweet chocolate, chopped (about ¼ cup)
    1 tablespoon half-and-half
    2 tablespoons ground flaxseed
    1 tablespoon slivered almonds, crushed or roughly chopped

Spread out the pretzels, orange sections, and strawberries on a large sheet of waxed paper. Place the chocolate and half-and-half in a small saucepan. Warm over low heat, stirring constantly, until the chocolate is smooth and completely melted.

With a rubber spatula, smooth the chocolate mixture over the pretzels and fruit slices. Sprinkle with the ground flaxseed and almonds. Let the chocolate cool 5 minutes, then transfer the tray to the refrigerator. Chill 15 to 20 minutes, until the chocolate is firm to the touch. Serve immediately or store in the fridge in an airtight container for 3 to 4 days.

Per serving (1 pretzel, 2 orange slices, or 1 strawberry):
60 calories, 1 g protein, 9 g carbohydrates, 3.1 g fat
(1.1 g saturated), 0 mg cholesterol, 1 g fiber, 10 mg sodium

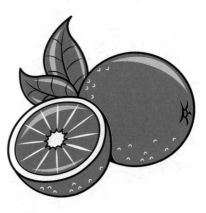

Frozen Fruit Skewers

SERVES 4

This recipe is inspired by ambrosia, a salad I used to enjoy as a child, only my version omits the customary marshmallows, which happen to contain high fructose corn syrup. Cut the tips off sharp skewers if you're serving this as a kids' dessert.

- 1 small mango (about 15 ounces), peeled and cut into 1-inch cubes
- 1 small banana (about 5 ounces), cut into 1-inch-thick slices
- 8 white or red grapes
- 8 raspberries, blackberries, or pitted cherries
- 4 12-inch wooden skewers
- ¼ cup reduced-fat sour cream
- ¼ cup chopped pecans
- ¼ cup sweetened coconut flakes

Thread the fruit onto the skewers, alternating between mango, banana, grapes, and berries. Using a rubber spatula, smear the fruit skewers with the sour cream. Sprinkle with the chopped pecans and coconut. Wrap the skewers in waxed paper, then transfer to a large zipper-lock bag and freeze 1 hour or more until firm.

Per serving (1 skewer): 202 calories, 2.3 g protein, 32 g carbohydrates, 8.9 g fat (2.9 g saturated), 6 mg cholesterol, 4 g fiber, 22 mg sodium

Chocolate Pudding Pops

MAKES 8 POPS

A lot of frozen treats on the market are low in sugar and fat, but what about all those preservatives and artificial sweeteners they contain? I'd rather eat the real thing. This frozen treat is lightened naturally with fat-free milk and the sweet flavor of carrot juice.

- 2 cups fat-free milk
- 1 cup carrot juice
- ¼ cup unsweetened cocoa powder
- 3 tablespoons granulated sugar
- 4 teaspoons cornstarch
- 2 teaspoons vanilla extract

Place the milk, carrot juice, cocoa, sugar, cornstarch, and vanilla in a large saucepan. Whisk briskly. Bring the mixture to slow boil, whisking continuously, until small bubbles start to form around the edges and the mixture is thick, 3 to 4 minutes. Transfer the mixture to 8 popsicle molds or paper drinking cups. Cover and freeze 3 to 4 hours or until firm. If using the paper cups, insert popsicle sticks after about 1 hour. Store in a freezer for up to 1 week.

Per serving (1 pop): 62 calories, 3 g protein, 12 g carbohydrates, 0.5 g fat (0 g saturated), 1 mg cholesterol, 1 g fiber, 45 mg sodium

Cherry Sherbet

SERVES 8

I'm a huge fan of frozen cherries because they are inexpensive, available year-round, and already pitted—and they taste simply delicious! Buttermilk adds texture and tartness to this sherbet, making this recipe a fast way to get an extra serving of fruit and satisfy your sweet tooth!

1 10-ounce bag frozen cherries
2 cups low-fat (1 percent) buttermilk
¼ cup reduced-fat cream cheese
6 tablespoons granulated sugar
1 tablespoon vanilla extract

Place all ingredients in a blender or food processor and process until smooth. Transfer the mixture to an airtight container and freeze 3 hours or more, until firm. Store in the freezer for up to 1 week.

Per serving (½ cup): 105 calories, 3 g protein, 19 g carbohydrates, 1.8 g fat (1 g saturated), 7 mg cholesterol, 1 g fiber, 101 mg sodium

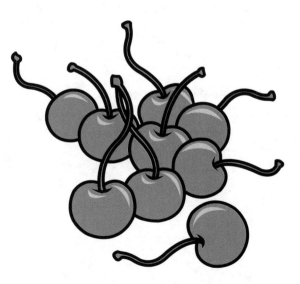

Frozen Coconut Yogurt

SERVES 8

The creamy texture of this treat tastes positively naughty—but it isn't! Once unfrozen, the yogurt also makes a great topping for fruit. Since yogurt is low in fat, this treat freezes hard, so let it defrost 1 hour on the countertop before you enjoy it. Or freeze in paper cups with popsicle sticks inserted to create a healthy frozen dessert on a stick!

$\frac{1}{2}$ cup unsweetened coconut flakes

4 cups (32 ounces) plain, fat-free Greek yogurt

$\frac{1}{2}$ cup confectioners' sugar

2 tablespoons ground flaxseed

1 tablespoon coconut extract

2 teaspoons vanilla extract

Preheat the oven to 350°F. Cover a small cookie sheet with aluminum foil. Spread the coconut on the sheet and bake 2 to 3 minutes, stirring once, until the coconut has lightly browned. Place the coconut in a large bowl with the yogurt, sugar, flaxseed, coconut extract, and vanilla. Whisk until smooth and transfer into a freezer-safe container. Freeze 1 hour or more until firm.

Per serving ($\frac{1}{2}$ cup): 147 calories, 11 g protein, 14 g carbohydrates, 4.4 g fat (3 g saturated), 0 mg cholesterol, 1 g fiber, 45 mg sodium

Vanilla Bean "Ice Cream"

SERVES 8

This treat, speckled with vanilla seeds, tastes as rich as ice cream made from heavy cream. If you don't have an ice-cream maker, you can freeze this dessert in an airtight container, such as a zipper-lock bag, stirring occasionally as it freezes.

½ cup packed brown sugar
3 egg yolks
2 cups fat-free milk
½ vanilla bean, cut in half and seeds scraped
1 cup plain, fat-free Greek yogurt

Fill a large bowl with ice. Place the sugar and egg yolks in another large bowl and whisk until smooth. Combine the milk and the vanilla bean pod and its seeds in a small saucepan; bring to a simmer. Transfer ½ cup of the warmed milk to the sugar mixture, immediately whisking until smooth. Repeat until all the milk has been incorporated smoothly into the sugar and egg mixture. Place the bowl directly into the large bowl of ice and allow the mixture to cool about 30 minutes. When the milk mixture is cool to the touch, whisk in the yogurt. Discard the vanilla pod. Transfer the liquid to an ice-cream maker and process according to the machine's instructions.

Per serving (½ cup): 110 calories, 6 g protein, 18 g carbohydrates, 1.7 g fat (0.6 g saturated), 79 mg cholesterol, 0 g fiber, 50 mg sodium

Hot Fudge Sundaes with Vanilla Bean Frozen Yogurt

SERVES 6

When you make a sundae yourself, you can control the amount of fat and sugar without losing that great combination of cold ice cream and hot chocolaty sauce.

 1 vanilla bean

 1 cup fat-free Greek yogurt

 1 15-ounce can peaches or apricots packed in water, drained

 ½ cup granulated sugar

 3 ripe bananas

 6 tablespoons chocolate sauce, heated

Cut the vanilla bean in half and scrape out the seeds. Place the seeds, yogurt, peaches or apricots, and sugar in a blender or food processor. Process until smooth. Transfer to a small freezer-safe container and freeze at least 3 hours or more, until firm.

Cut the bananas lengthwise in half and remove the peels. Cut each banana in half crosswise. Place 2 banana quarters into each of 6 small dishes or wine glasses. Spoon two small scoops of the frozen yogurt in between the slices of banana. Drizzle with the chocolate sauce and serve immediately.

Per serving (½ cup yogurt + ½ banana + 1 tablespoon chocolate sauce): 166 calories, 4 g protein, 34 g carbohydrates, 1.7 g fat (0.7 g saturated), 0 mg cholesterol, 1 g fiber, 81 mg sodium

SKINNY SHOPPING LIST

Want to start eating healthier right away? Stock your fridge, freezer, and pantry with healthy staples that can be used for all kind of recipes—here are the ingredients you'd find if you were cooking in my kitchen! Think of this as your weekly shopping checklist for everything you'll need to start on the path to a healthier you.

The more whole unprocessed foods you buy—like fresh vegetables, fruits, lean meats, and low-fat dairy and whole grains—the healthier your shopping cart will be. It's always good to have a small snack before you hit the grocery store to avoid crazy "impulse" buying. Shopping with kids? Let them know that they can pick out the ingredients to make one dessert for the week and as you walk the aisles, jot down or call out their own "mini" shopping list to keep them focused on shopping for quality ingredients instead of reaching for junk food.

Fridge

DAIRY

- ☐ Half-and-half
- ☐ Low-fat (1 percent) buttermilk
- ☐ Skim milk
- ☐ Reduced-fat and fat-free sour cream
- ☐ Plain, fat-free Greek yogurt
- ☐ Reduced-fat cream cheese
- ☐ Parmesan cheese
- ☐ Part-skim mozzarella cheese
- ☐ Part-skim and fat-free ricotta cheese
- ☐ Reduced-fat (2 percent) Cheddar cheese
- ☐ Reduced-fat Swiss cheese
- ☐ Butter
- ☐ Trans-fat-free margarine
- ☐ Eggs

MEAT

- ☐ Bone-in chicken breasts, skin removed
- ☐ Skinless, boneless chicken breasts
- ☐ Ground turkey
- ☐ Nitrate-free turkey bacon
- ☐ Turkey sausage
- ☐ Trimmed beef sirloin
- ☐ Center-cut pork chops
- ☐ Low-sodium sliced ham

CRISPER

- ☐ Apples
- ☐ Blueberries
- ☐ Strawberries
- ☐ Lemons
- ☐ Limes
- ☐ Oranges
- ☐ Baby spinach
- ☐ Broccoli
- ☐ Carrots
- ☐ Cauliflower
- ☐ Celery
- ☐ Cucumbers
- ☐ Jalapeño peppers
- ☐ Mushrooms
- ☐ Red and green bell peppers
- ☐ Romaine lettuce
- ☐ Scallions
- ☐ Zucchini
- ☐ Basil
- ☐ Cilantro
- ☐ Flat-leaf parsley
- ☐ Thyme

OTHER

- ☐ Carrot juice
- ☐ Orange juice
- ☐ Ground flaxseed

Freezer

- ☐ Frozen cherries
- ☐ Peas
- ☐ Phyllo

Pantry

- ☐ Canola oil
- ☐ Nonstick cooking spray
- ☐ Olive oil
- ☐ Brown rice or multigrain pasta
- ☐ Quinoa
- ☐ Rolled old-fashioned oats
- ☐ Short-grain brown rice
- ☐ White whole wheat flour
- ☐ Whole wheat angel hair pasta
- ☐ Whole wheat baguette
- ☐ Whole wheat bread crumbs
- ☐ Whole wheat bread or whole grain bread
- ☐ Whole wheat pita
- ☐ Whole wheat or whole grain tortillas
- ☐ Whole wheat tortilla chips
- ☐ Canned black beans
- ☐ Canned chickpeas
- ☐ Canned chipotle chiles

☐ Canned kidney beans

☐ Reduced-sodium beef broth

☐ Reduced-sodium, fat-free chicken
    broth

☐ Reduced-sodium soy sauce

☐ Jarred pickled jalapeño peppers

☐ Jarred tomato sauce

☐ Tomato paste

☐ Whole peeled tomatoes

☐ Balsamic vinegar

☐ Dijon mustard

☐ Hot sauce

☐ Reduced-fat mayonnaise

☐ Bittersweet chocolate chips

☐ Brown sugar

☐ Granulated sugar

☐ Honey

☐ Maple syrup

☐ Prunes

☐ Raisins

☐ Reduced-fat peanut butter

☐ Unsweetened cocoa powder

☐ Vanilla extract

☐ Walnuts

SPICES

☐ Black pepper

☐ Cayenne pepper

☐ Curry powder

☐ Garlic powder

☐ Ground cinnamon

☐ Ground cumin

☐ Mild chili powder

☐ Nutmeg

☐ Onion powder

☐ Paprika

☐ Star anise

☐ Taco seasoning without MSG

COUNTERTOP

☐ Avocados

☐ Bananas

☐ Garlic

☐ Onions

☐ Sweet potatoes

☐ Tomatoes

☐ White potatoes

RECIPE INDEX BY CATEGORY

SCHOOL OR WORK LUNCH

Alarmingly Good Low-Fat Chili, page 34

Baked "Deep Fried" Chicken with Crunchy Double Whole Grain Breading, page 68

Baked Meatballs with Zesty Marinara, page 86

Banana Bread, page 150

"Cream" of Broccoli Soup with Cheddar, page 36

Four Food Groups Minestrone, page 32

Garlicky Black Bean Soup, page 30

Light Lasagna Made with Turkey and Veggies, page 54

Meatball Sandwiches, page 88

Mock Crab Cakes with Zucchini and Tuna, page 64

Slender Blondie Brownies with Walnuts, Chocolate Chips, and Prunes, page 146

Stuffed Peppers Cooked in Pepperoni-Flavored Tomato Sauce, page 58

Stuffed Shells That Won't Leave You Feeling Stuffed, page 56

Ten-Minute Chicken Noodle Soup, page 38

Zucchini Bread Fit for Breakfast, Too, page 152

KID FRIENDLY

Alarmingly Good Low-Fat Chili, page 34

Baked "Deep Fried" Chicken with Crunchy Double Whole Grain Breading, page 68

Baked Meatballs with Zesty Marinara, page 86

Baked Steak House Fries, page 103

Banana Bread, page 150

Banana Cream Pie, page 132

Carrot Cake with Applesauce and Carrot Juice, page 136

Chocolate Pudding Pops, page 157

Four Food Groups Minestrone, page 32

Garlicky Black Bean Soup, page 30

Good Lookin' Grilled Cheese, page 57

Just Like Takeout Sweet-and-Sour Chicken, page 72

Light Lasagna Made with Turkey and Veggies, page 54

Mac and Cheese with Shredded Chicken and Cauliflower, page 52

Meatball Sandwiches, page 88

Pork Lo Mein, Hold the Grease, page 92

Ricotta Strawberry Shortcake Parfaits, page 154

Sesame Chicken Hold the Deep-Fried Breading, page 74

Slender Blondie Brownies with Walnuts, Chocolate Chips, and Prunes, page 146

Spicy Sloppy Joes with Carrot and Red Bell Pepper, page 94

Stuffed Chicken Parmesan, page 66

Stuffed Shells That Won't Leave You Feeling Stuffed, page 58

Supermoist Turkey Burgers, page 82

Tantalizing Turkey Tacos with Star Anise, page 84

Ten-Minute Chicken Noodle Soup, page 38

EASY TO COOK WITH KIDS

Almond Dressing, page 119

Bacon-Wrapped Dates, page 40

Blender Pancakes with Sweet Cinnamon Bananas, page 10

Carrot Ginger Dressing, page 118

Creamy Mexican Bean Dip with Whole Grain Tortilla Chips, page 41

Party Mix with Spiced Nuts and Whole Grain Cereal, page 46

Peanut Butter Spread and Jelly on Toast, page 20

Poolside Soup, page 39

ONE-POT MEALS AND DESSERT FOR POTLUCKS

Alarmingly Good Low-Fat Chili, page 34

Banana Cream Pie, page 132

Blueberry Cobbler with Yogurt Topping, page 134

Carrot Cake with Applesauce and Carrot Juice, page 136

Chicken and Rice Hot Pot, page 76

Chicken "No Pot Belly" Pie, page 70

Crustless Apple Pie, page 131

Italian Cheesecake, page 143

Light Lasagna Made with Turkey and Veggies, page 54

My Dad's Trim Chicken Enchiladas, page 67

Scalloped Potatoes with Ham, page 105

HOLIDAYS

Winter

Almond Dressing, page 119

Baked Meatballs with Zesty Marinara, page 86

Butternut Squash Soup with Coconut Milk, page 27

Honey-Roasted Baby Carrots with Raisins, page 121

Italian Cheesecake, page 143

Scalloped Potatoes with Ham, page 105

Shrimp and Corn Chowder, page 37

Sinful Chocolate Cake Made with Raisins and Bittersweet Morsels, page 142

Stuffed Peppers Cooked in Pepperoni-Flavored Tomato Sauce, page 58

Stuffed Shells That Won't Leave You Feeling Stuffed, page 56

Spring

Bacon Spinach Salad, page 116

Banana Cream Pie, page 132

Mock Crab Cakes with Zucchini and Tuna, page 64

Rainbow Macaroni Salad with Tuna, page 60

Ricotta Strawberry Shortcake Parfaits, page 154

Three Bean Salad, page 114

Summer

Banana Bread, page 150

Blueberry Cobbler with Yogurt Topping, page 134

Broccoli Bacon Salad, page 113

Buttermilk Yogurt Dressing, page 117

Carrot Ginger Dressing, page 118

Cucumber Salad with Sour Cream and Fresh Dill, page 115

Mock Crab Cakes with Zucchini and Tuna, page 64

My Granny's Cinnamon Coffee Cake the Skinny Way, page 140

Rainbow Macaroni Salad with Tuna, page 60

Ricotta Strawberry Shortcake Parfaits, page 154

Three Bean Salad, page 114

Zucchini Bread Fit for Breakfast, Too, page 152

Fall

Carrot Cake with Applesauce and Carrot Juice, page 136

Green Beans with Almonds and Lemon Pepper Croutons, page 120

Honey-Roasted Baby Carrots with Raisins, page 121

My Granny's Cinnamon Coffee Cake the Skinny Way, page 140

Sinful Chocolate Cake Made with Raisins and Bittersweet Morsels, page 142

Slender Blondie Brownies with Walnuts, Chocolate Chips, and Prunes, page 146

Zucchini Bread Fit for Breakfast, Too, page 152

FINGER FOOD FOR FOOTBALL GAMES AND PARTIES

Bacon-Wrapped Dates, page 40

Banana Bread, page 150

Chocolate-Covered Pretzels and Fruit, page 155

Creamy Mexican Bean Dip with Whole Grain Tortilla Chips, page 41

Frozen Fruit Skewers, page 156

Hot "Wings" with Spicy Sauce, page 44

Meatball Sandwiches, page 88

Nachos Grande with Pickled Jalapeño Salsa, page 42

Party Dip Served with Whole Wheat Pita, page 45

Party Mix with Spiced Nuts and Whole Grain Cereal, page 46

Slender Blondie Brownies with Walnuts, Chocolate Chips, and Prunes, page 146

Stuffed Mushrooms with Blue Cheese, page 107

WORK OUT BEFORE AND AFTER

Chocolate Breakfast Shake, page 22

"Cream" of Broccoli Soup with Cheddar, page 36

Essential Smoothie, page 23

French Tuna Salad, page 62

Garlicky Black Bean Soup, page 30

Poolside Soup, page 39

Seven-Minute Salmon, page 65

BRUNCH

Apple Butter, page 21

Bacon Sausage Omelet with Onions and Peppers, page 4

Baked "Deep Fried" Chicken with Crunchy Double Whole Grain Breading, page 68

Blender Pancakes with Sweet Cinnamon Bananas, page 10

Blueberry Cobbler with Yogurt Topping, page 134

Buttermilk Biscuits, page 125

French Toast with Orange Marmalade, page 16

French Tuna Salad, page 62

Lemony Yogurt Muffins, page 18

Maple Apple Waffles, page 14

Mock Crab Cakes with Zucchini and Tuna, page 64

My Dad's Trim Chicken Enchiladas, page 67

Zucchini Pancakes with Walnuts and Spice, page 12

RESTAURANT FAVORITES YOU CAN MAKE AT HOME

Baked Steak House Fries, page 103

Breaded Zucchini with Marinara Dipping Sauce, page 108

Chicken Marsala with Mushrooms and Broccoli, page 80

French Onion Soup with Cheesy Whole Wheat Croutons, page 28

Garlicky Black Bean Soup, page 30

Hot "Wings" with Spicy Sauce, page 44

Just Like Takeout Sweet-and-Sour Chicken, page 72

Pork Lo Mein, Hold the Grease, page 92

Sesame Chicken Hold the Deep-Fried Breading, page 74

Shrimp and Corn Chowder, page 37

Steak and Potatoes, page 96

Supermoist Turkey Burgers, page 82

THROW A TAPAS OR COCKTAIL PARTY

Bacon-Wrapped Dates, page 40

Breaded Zucchini with Marinara Dipping Sauce, page 108

Hot "Wings" with Spicy Sauce, page 44

Mock Crab Cakes with Zucchini and Tuna, page 64

Ricotta Strawberry Shortcake Parfaits, page 154

Shrimp and Corn Fritters, page 110

Stuffed Mushrooms with Blue Cheese, page 107

SUPERFAST WEEKNIGHT MEALS

Bacon Spinach Salad, page 116

Cut the Fat, Keep the Creamy Pasta Carbonara, page 51

Good Lookin' Grilled Cheese, page 57

Mock Crab Cakes with Zucchini and Tuna, page 64

Ricotta Strawberry Shortcake Parfaits, page 154

Seven-Minute Salmon, page 65

Simple Sautéed Spinach with Garlic and Chile Flakes, page 122

Spicy Sloppy Joes with Carrot and Red Bell Pepper, page 94

Stir-Fried Garlic Broccoli, page 123

Tantalizing Turkey Tacos with Star Anise, page 84

Ten-Minute Chicken Noodle Soup, page 38

Warm Creamed Spinach Minus the Heavy Cream, page 124

ROMANTIC DINNERS FOR TWO

Apple Strudel with Walnut Crumble Topping, page 148

Bacon Spinach Salad, page 116

Banana Bread, page 150

Blueberry Cobbler with Yogurt Topping, page 134

Broccoli Bacon Salad, page 113

Buttermilk Yogurt Dressing, page 117

Butternut Squash Soup with Coconut Milk, page 27

Carrot Cake with Applesauce and Carrot Juice, page 136

Carrot Ginger Dressing, page 118

Cherry Sherbet, page 158

Chicken Marsala with Mushrooms and Broccoli, page 80

Chocolate-Covered Pretzels and Fruit, page 155

Cucumber Salad with Sour Cream and Fresh Dill, page 115

Cut the Fat, Keep the Creamy Pasta Carbonara, page 51

French Onion Soup with Cheesy Whole Wheat Croutons, page 28

French Tuna Salad, page 62

Frozen Coconut Yogurt, page 159

Frozen Fruit Skewers, page 156

Hot Fudge Sundaes with Vanilla Bean Frozen Yogurt, page 161

Mock Crab Cakes with Zucchini and Tuna, page 64

Seven-Minute Salmon, page 65

Shrimp and Corn Chowder, page 37

Steak and Potatoes, page 96

Stuffed Chicken Parmesan, page 66

Stuffed Peppers Cooked in Pepperoni-Flavored Tomato Sauce, page 58

Vanilla Bean "Ice Cream," page 160

Warm Creamed Spinach Minus the Heavy Cream, page 124

SUBSTITUTIONS

Safe for Celiac Disease

These recipes are safe for people with celiac disease, as long as you buy the "wheat free" versions of ingredients such as soy sauce, pasta sauce, etc.

Alarmingly Good Low-Fat Chili, page 34

Almond Dressing, page 119

Apple Butter, page 21

Bacon Sausage Omelet with Onions and Peppers, page 4

Bacon Spinach Salad, page 116

Bacon-Wrapped Dates, page 40

Baked Eggs and Ham, page 6

Baked Steak House Fries, page 103

Broccoli Bacon Salad, page 113

Buttermilk Yogurt Dressing, page 117

Butternut Squash Soup with Coconut Milk, page 27

Carrot Ginger Dressing, page 118

Cherry Sherbet, page 158

Chocolate Breakfast Shake, page 22

Chocolate Pudding Pops, page 157

"Cream" of Broccoli Soup with Cheddar, page 36

Cucumber Salad with Sour Cream and Fresh Dill, page 115

Essential Smoothie, page 23

French Tuna Salad, page 62

Frozen Coconut Yogurt, page 159

Honey-Roasted Baby Carrots with Raisins, page 121

Hot Fudge Sundaes with Vanilla Bean Frozen Yogurt, page 161

Hot "Wings" with Spicy Sauce, page 44

"Mayonnaise Is Not Your Enemy" Coleslaw, page 112

Pigs in a Blanket, page 90

Poolside Soup, page 39

Rainbow Macaroni Salad with Tuna, page 60

Sesame Chicken Hold the Deep-Fried Breading, page 74

Seven-Minute Salmon, page 65

Shrimp and Corn Chowder, page 37

Simple Sautéed Spinach with Garlic and Chile Flakes, page 122

Southwestern Frittata with Spicy Corn Salsa, page 8

Stir-Fried Garlic Broccoli, page 123

Stuffed Peppers Cooked in Pepperoni-Flavored Tomato Sauce, page 58

Tantalizing Turkey Tacos with Star Anise, page 84

Three Bean Salad, page 114

Twice-Baked Potatoes with Filling So Rich No One Will Know It's Low Fat, page 104

Vanilla Bean "Ice Cream," page 160

Substitute Brown Rice Pasta to Make These Recipes Celiac Safe as well

Cut the Fat, Keep the Creamy Pasta Carbonara, page 51

Four Food Groups Minestrone, page 32

Ten-Minute Chicken Noodle Soup, page 38

I'll admit it, there are nights when even I don't feel like cooking. It doesn't happen often, but when it does, I go for something fast and nutritious: a real meal instead of a bagel or a bag of chips. Here are a few tips for creating tasty and highly nutritious salads, snacks, and hot meals when you don't feel like making a big deal out of dinner.

Making a Salad into a Real Meal

Salads are the single most misunderstood "healthy" meals. Dressing is the most common subject of debate: Is the dressing good or bad? Is it fatty or high in sugar? Is cream-based dressing a no-no? What exactly does "xantham gum" mean? (It's a food stabilizer, by the way, meaning that it keeps the dressing from separating.) While it is important to check the nutrition label of any purchased dressing so that you enjoy a reasonably low-fat and low-calorie dressing, it can be just as easy to make your own dressing that exactly fits your taste!

As you probably know, salad dressings can be one of those "fat traps"—a salad with 4 tablespoons of dressing can have more fat than a juicy hamburger! The best way to dress your salad is to turn to a low-fat dressing recipe with fresh ingredients that aren't loaded with preservatives. I love fat-free yogurt, lemon, herbs, fresh ginger, garlic, and a little olive oil as building blocks.

I don't believe in eating a fat-free diet. Our bodies need some fat to feel full and to absorb fat-soluble vitamins like A, D, and K. Although some fat is fine in your dressing, it's important to not go overboard and needlessly double up on calories. Here are three options that are fast, tasty, and naturally fat free:

- 2 tablespoons jarred tomato salsa, mild or spicy
- Juice of half a fresh lemon (or lime), plus a pinch of salt
- 1 tablespoon honey mixed with 1 tablespoon mustard and 1 teaspoon vinegar

If you decide to select a fat-free dressing, you can pick from one of the following add-ins to add lots of flavor and just a little fat to help you feel full:

- 4 to 5 almonds, chopped
- 1 tablespoon blue cheese
- 1 slice cooked bacon, crumbled
- 1 tablespoon sliced olives
- ¼ ripe avocado, diced

Beyond using healthy salad dressings, the real art to making a tasty salad is to create it the right way: Salads can be especially beneficial if you choose vegetables that provide extra vitamins and vital nutrients that we all need for healthy and gorgeous bodies.

Not all lettuces are created equal. Iceburg lettuce, while crunchy and refreshing, doesn't contain much in the way of vitamins and minerals. You can still enjoy it by mixing in other vegetables, but if you want a real power base for your salad—that will also make a complete meal—pick one of these choices:

- **Baby spinach.** Baby spinach is my number one choice because spinach has vitamin and mineral power, from vitamin C to folate. Having trouble seeing without your glasses? Just 1 cup of fresh spinach contains over 300 percent of your daily needs for vitamin A for healthy eyes.

- **Romaine lettuce.** Want your bones to be strong? Wish to see cuts and bruises heal faster? Then get your romaine on! Just 2 cups give you 140 percent of your daily needs for vitamin K.

- **Mixed baby greens.** Prewashed baby greens can be convenient and tasty. Baby mixed greens typically contain beet greens, spinach, romaine, and a whole host of superveggies (check the ingredients list before you buy). To be sure you're getting a good brand, take a peek at the nutrition label: If you see high percentages for things like vitamin A, vitamin C, and iron, then you've got one for your fridge!

Lean protein is the best way to satisfy a hearty appetite, and you should consider adding some to your salad. Here's why: Even if you're not a big eater, a lean protein like fish, chicken, and turkey will help keep your blood sugar levels even and will keep late-night snack cravings away! This will make it much easier to maintain or reach your healthy weight.

Fast No-Mess Meals for One

Eating pasta all the time gets old. Keeping your meals fresh and interesting can help you to maintain or even lose weight as well as ensure richer nutrition by using varied healthy ingredients. Here are some quick ideas when you've only got about 15 minutes to spare and still crave a hot meal.

Fresh Veggie Stir-Fry

Take ¼ head of broccoli and roughly chop it, then add in a handful of sliced mushrooms and bell pepper. Heat a large skillet with 1 teaspoon of olive oil, add the veggies, and sprinkle with salt. Cook until the veggies are tender crisp, 6 to 8 minutes. Enjoy your veggie stir-fry with a tablespoon of barbecue sauce, teriyaki sauce, or low-fat salad dressing. Round it out with a small toasted pita.

Hot from the Freezer

I always keep a bag of precooked shrimp in my freezer, along with packages of frozen veggies that don't lose their nutrition as quickly as fresh produce. My favorite is the broccoli-cauliflower-carrot mix. Just heat 1 teaspoon of olive oil in a large skillet and add 2 cups of your frozen veggie mix. Add a few tablespoons of water, cover, and cook 4 to 5 minutes, until the vegetables are warm. Toss in a few cooked shrimp, sprinkle with a little salt, then add hot sauce and ¼ cup pasta sauce. Cook an additional minute to warm the sauce.

Sausage and Peppers

Combine vegetables with slices of a cooked good-quality, nitrate-free chicken sausage and you can have a fast, filling meal in minutes. Just heat a large skillet over high heat with 1 teaspoon of olive oil and add a handful of raw broccoli florets along with ½ cup of thinly sliced red bell pepper. After the vegetables begin to soften (2 to 3 minutes), add a few tablespoons of water and cover. Cook another minute, until the veggies are crisp but tender. Add the sausage slices and 1 cup of spinach; cook 1 more minute, until the sausage is warm and the spinach wilts. Round out your meal with a few whole wheat crackers or a small slice of whole wheat bread.

Quesadilla

A delicious, healthy quesadilla starts with a soft whole wheat wrap. Add a protein boost with 1 slice of lean lunch meat—such as low-sodium ham or roasted turkey—and then tuck in fast-cooking veggies such as mushrooms, roasted red bell peppers, baby spinach, thinly sliced tomato, or 1 cup of mashed black beans or navy beans. Top with ¼ cup shredded part-skim mozzarella, then toast your quesadilla in the oven for 10 minutes at 400°F, or in a dry skillet for 4 to 5 minutes over medium heat, turning once or twice.

Not Your Average Healthy Snack

What do you think of when you hear "healthy snack"? Do you think nuts, seeds, dried fruit, granola bar, or yogurt? Well, if you don't read the nutrition labels on snack packaging, you could be in for quite a shock: Many of those so-called healthy snacks can pack in loads of fat and calories. The best healthy snack starts with vegetables and fresh fruit. Here are some ideas, and you don't have to be a chef or a nutritionist to prepare them.

- 1 medium apple coated with 1 tablespoon reduced-fat peanut butter
- 1 cup red grapes and 3 whole wheat crackers with 1 wedge (0.75 ounce) reduced-fat cheese spread, such as Laughing Cow
- Handful of carrots or raw broccoli florets dipped in 1 tablespoon of your favorite barbecue sauce
- Cut the sugar in half by skipping those ultrasugary "fruit on the bottom" yogurts. Instead, go for 1 small container of plain, fat-free yogurt—I love Greek yogurt!—and add one of these choices:

    1 tablespoon bittersweet chocolate chips

    2 teaspoons honey

    2 tablespoons applesauce

    1 small biscotto, crumbled

    ¼ cup frozen black cherries

    ½ medium banana, thinly sliced

HOW TO USE LEFTOVERS

Why throw away good food? Learn how to use that last carrot at the bottom of the crisper, and you'll save money and eat well.

How to Use Leftovers of Recipes in this Book

Southwestern Frittata with Spicy Corn Salsa, page 8

This is one egg dish that holds up to being refrigerated. I just set leftovers on the counter to let it come to room temperature. You can tuck a slice into a pita and add a slice of tomato and a few fresh spinach leaves and voilà, a fast lunch.

Blender Pancakes, page 10

This is a fantastic recipe for entertaining. You can fill them with savory fillings: I like to place a slice of ham and low-fat Swiss between two pancakes and heat them in a skillet. You can also fill them with sautéed mushrooms and a dollop of goat cheese, then serve with a salad, for a whole meal.

Maple Apple Waffles, page 14

Leftovers are great to pack in a school lunch for a savory or sweet treat. To make a sandwich, cut one waffle in half, smear a teaspoon of low-fat cream cheese on each half, and add two slices of roast turkey and a piece of romaine lettuce. To make a great dessert, simply cut one waffle in half on the diagonal, spread 2 tablespoons of low-fat store-bought pudding on one side, and top with the other half.

Alarmingly Good Low-Fat Chili, page 34

Ok, so you only have a cup of the chili left over—not enough for a whole meal. Don't toss it, use it as taco filling, topping it with grated part-skim mozzarella, chopped baby spinach or romaine, and chopped tomatoes. Add taco sauce and lunch is ready. For a more gourmet option, take store-bought roasted red peppers, fill each with chili, and top with salsa and shredded part-skim mozzarella. Bake for 10 minutes at 400°F, until the cheese is hot and bubbly.

"Cream" of Broccoli Soup with Cheddar, page 16

Everyone knows the old "top the baked potato" trick. But this leftover soup can also be used as a sauce for stuffed leftover Blender Pancakes, page 10. Just cook a large package of sliced white mushrooms with a little olive oil and garlic, mix with low-fat or fat-free ricotta off the heat, and roll the filling in the crepes. Top with soup and sprinkle a little shredded part-skim mozzarella over it.

Creamy Mexican Bean Dip with Whole Grain Tortilla Chips, page 41

Who feels like cooking a huge meal the day after a party? Leftover bean dip makes an excellent filling for quesadillas. Just smear one side of a soft whole grain tortilla with a little dip, top with baby spinach, thinly sliced mushrooms, and a little chopped red onion. Sprinkle with 2 table-spoons of your favorite low-fat cheese and top with another tortilla. Heat a large skillet with nonstick spray and brown each side for 1 to 2 minutes.

Hot "Wings" with Spicy Sauce, page 44

I guarantee there won't be any chicken left over when you make this, but you might have a bit of the sauce. You can toss the spicy sauce with pasta, roasted red peppers, and cooked shrimp, and top with grated Parmesan to make a fast "Diavolo" sauce.

Stuffed Peppers Cooked in Pepperoni-Flavored Tomato Sauce, page 58

Stuffed peppers are a great meal for hearty appetites, but usually there is a little sauce left over. Don't dump the flavorful, rich tasting sauce down the drain, use it to top a simple seared chicken breast, or serve alongside Breaded Zucchini with Marinara Dipping Sauce, page 108, in place of the marinara.

Chicken Marsala with Mushrooms and Broccoli, page 80

I know this is a classic Italian dish, but you can chop up leftovers and heat in a skillet with a little brown rice for a fried rice dish. When the mixture is hot, push it to the side. Add one beaten egg to the empty space and cook 1 minute until the egg starts to set. Stir once or twice to incorporate and serve with a handful of chopped scallions.

Seven-Minute Salmon, page 65

Fish doesn't keep very well as a leftover, but salmon can be tasty if used the very next day. If you make this for a dinner party on Friday, add leftovers to your Saturday morning omelet along with a handful of arugula or baby spinach.

Baked "Deep Fried" Chicken with Crunchy Double Whole Grain Breading, page 68

The breading stays on this chicken, even after it cools, which makes it perfectly portable. Slice and use as a topping for a workplace salad or pack with a little honey mustard for your little one's school lunch along with carrot sticks and a piece of fruit.

Chicken and Rice Hot Pot, page 76

I'm sure you have at least one person in your family who will eat the top of the pie and leave half the filling underneath! Don't toss the filling—it reheats nicely and can be served with a half cup of whole grain pasta or brown rice.

Spicy Sloppy Joes with Carrot and Red Bell Pepper, page 94

Kids love the taste of flavorful ground meat. Make a personalized "sloppy pizza" by spreading the sloppy joe meat over a soft whole wheat tortilla and topping with 2 tablespoons of part-skim mozzarella. Bake at 400°F for 8 to 10 minutes until the cheese is bubbly.

How to Use Fridge Odds and Ends

One carrot at the bottom of the bag

Peel and grate the carrot on a box grater and stir into the tomato sauce for any of my Italian dishes: Stuffed Shells That Won't Leave You Feeling Stuffed, page 56; Light Lasagna Made with Turkey and Veggies, page 54; Stuffed Peppers Cooked in Pepperoni-Flavored Tomato Sauce, page 58; Baked Meatballs with Zesty Marinara, page 86; or Meatball Sandwiches, page 88.

One slice of turkey

If you're making the Bacon, Egg, and Cheese Sandwich, page 3, sub one slice of turkey for the bacon.

Handful of button mushrooms

Roughly chop by hand or in a food processor and mix into Supermoist Turkey Burgers, page 82.

Quarter cup of skim milk

Add to "Cream" of Broccoli Soup with Cheddar, page 36; Shrimp and Corn Chowder, page 37; or Butternut Squash Soup with Coconut Milk, page 27.

Scoop of low-fat ricotta

Substitute the ricotta for ½ cup of the milk in the Chocolate Breakfast Shake, page 22, or drizzle with a tablespoon of good-quality chocolate syrup for a satisfying little dessert.

Handful of broccoli florets

Roughly chop by hand or in a minichopper and mix into Baked Meatballs with Zesty Marinara, page 86.

Steamed brown rice

Plain steamed brown rice, even from takeout, will keep well overnight. Add it to any of these recipes for a complete meal: Tender Beef Stroganoff, page 98; Just Like Takeout Sweet-and-Sour Chicken, page 72; or Sesame Chicken Hold the Deep-Fried Breading, page 74.

ONLINE RESOURCES

Feeling too busy to figure out how to make my Skinny Secrets work for you? Tired of fighting with your kids about eating healthier foods?

I have produced five *free* resources to transition you effortlessly to a new eating and cooking approach that will bring lasting benefits and help keep your weight in check. Yes, you *can* have your cake and eat it too!

These resources, inspired by *Secrets of a Skinny Chef,* will help you put the book's principles into practice in your life.

Cook Like a Skinny Chef—Videos

You don't have to be a professionally trained chef to create delicious, mouthwatering meals that are also healthy. But if you rarely cook at home, watch these six videos—I demonstrate basic cooking techniques and explain unfamiliar concepts that you may come across in the recipes in this book.

Shop Like a Skinny Chef— Shopping and Product List

Eating healthier becomes easier when you know what groceries to purchase and how to stock your pantry. Download my skinny shopping list so you can take it with you to the grocery store and easily select nutritious foods.

Skinny Chef's Weekly Secrets

How about easy reminders of the book's key principles and secrets? Download the handy reference chart and hang it on your kitchen wall! Better yet, sign up for my weekly expert tips on making healthy changes stick permanently.

12 Secrets to Get Started—Quick-Start Booklet

Making changes can seem daunting, and convincing the rest of your family to adopt healthy habits might be tough. Download the *12 Skinny Chef Secrets to Kick Off Your New Lifestyle*—easy and simple changes that you can make today. Your taste buds (and your family) won't complain!

Becoming a Skinny Chef—Audio Lesson

Sick of dieting and yo-yoing weight? This audio lesson explains how I turned my childhood struggles into an eating and cooking philosophy that can work for everyone. Ditch your diets and enjoy decadent foods without guilt!

For these free resources and much more,
visit SecretsOfASkinnyChef.com/resources

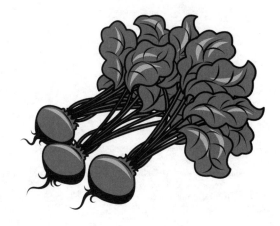

INDEX

Underscored page references indicate boxed text or tips. Page numbers followed by ★ indicate photographs in the color insert.

Almonds

adding to muffin recipe, 18
adding to salad dressing, 176
Almond Dressing, 119
Bacon-Wrapped Dates, 40
Chocolate-Covered Pretzels and Fruit, 155
Green Beans with Almonds and Lemon Pepper Croutons, 120
Party Mix with Spiced Nuts and Whole Grain Cereal, 46–47
Poolside Soup, 39

Appetizers

Bacon-Wrapped Dates, 40
Creamy Mexican Bean Dip with Whole Grain Tortilla Chips, 41
Hot "Wings" with Spicy Sauce, 44
Nachos Grande with Pickled Jalapeño Salsa, 42–43
Party Dip Served with Whole Wheat Pita, 45
Party Mix with Spiced Nuts and Whole Grain Cereal, 46–47

Apples

Apple Butter, 21
Apple Strudel with Walnut Crumble Topping, 148–49
Crustless Apple Pie, 131
Maple Apple Waffles, 14–15
"Mayonnaise Is Not Your Enemy" Coleslaw, 112

Applesauce

Carrot Cake with Applesauce and Carrot Juice, 136–37
as oil substitute in desserts, 137
Tiramisu Parfaits, 144–45★

Apricots

Hot Fudge Sundae with Vanilla Bean Frozen Yogurt, 161
as oil substitute in desserts, 137
Arteriosclerosis, xxi

Artichokes

Party Dip Served with Whole Wheat Pita, 45

Asian-style dishes

Carrot Ginger Dressing, 118
Just Like Takeout Sweet-and-Sour Chicken, 72–73★
Pork Lo Mein, Hold the Grease, 92–93
Sesame Chicken Hold the Deep-Fried Breading, 74–75
Seven-Minute Salmon, 65
Stir-Fried Garlic Broccoli, 123

Avocados

adding to salad dressing, 176
French Tuna Salad, 62–63
Nachos Grande with Pickled Jalapeño Salsa, 42–43
Poolside Soup, 39

Bacon, turkey

adding to salad dressing, 176
Bacon, Egg, and Cheese Sandwich, 3
Bacon Sausage Omelet with Onions and Peppers, 4–5
Bacon Spinach Salad, 116
Bacon-Wrapped Dates, 40
benefits of, 3
Broccoli Bacon Salad, 113
Cut the Fat, Keep the Creamy Pasta Carbonara, 51
Shrimp and Corn Chowder, 37★
Twice-Baked Potatoes with Filling So Rich No One Will Know It's Low Fat, 104

Bamboo shoots

Just Like Takeout Sweet-and-Sour Chicken, 72–73★
Sesame Chicken Hold the Deep-Fried Breading, 74–75

Bananas

Banana Bread, 150–51
Banana Cream Pie, 132–33★
Blender Pancakes with Sweet Cinnamon Bananas, 10–11
Chocolate Angel Food Cupcakes with Angelic Icing, 138–39
Chocolate Breakfast Shake, 22
Essential Smoothie, 23
Frozen Fruit Skewers, 156
Hot Fudge Sundae with Vanilla Bean Frozen Yogurt, 161
as oil substitute in desserts, 137
Zucchini Pancakes with Walnuts and Spice, 12–13

Basil

Baked Eggs and Ham, 6
Buttermilk Yogurt Dressing, 117

Chicken and Rice Hot Pot, 76–77
Cut the Fat, Keep the Creamy Pasta Carbonara, 51
Four Food Groups Minestrone, 32–33
Good Lookin' Grilled Cheese, 57
health benefits, 6
Stuffed Peppers Cooked in Pepperoni-Flavored Tomato Sauce, 58–59
Supermoist Turkey Burgers, 82–83

Beans. See also Green beans

Alarmingly Good Low-Fat Chili, 34–35
Creamy Mexican Bean Dip with Whole Grain Tortilla Chips, 41
Four Food Groups Minestrone, 32–33
Garlicky Black Bean Soup, 30–31
Nachos Grande with Pickled Jalapeño Salsa, 42–43
Party Dip Served with Whole Wheat Pita, 45
Party Mix with Spiced Nuts and Whole Grain Cereal, 46–47
Southwestern Frittata with Spicy Corn Salsa, 8–9★
Tantalizing Turkey Tacos with Star Anise, 84–85
Three Bean Salad, 114

Beef

fillet mignon, cooking tip, 66
Four Food Groups Minestrone, 32–33
Pigs in a Blanket, 90–91
slicing, tip for, 99
Spicy Sloppy Joes with Carrot and Red Bell Pepper, 94–95
Steak and Potatoes, 96–97★
Tender Beef Stroganoff, 98–99

Bell peppers

Alarmingly Good Low-Fat Chili, 34–35
Bacon Sausage Omelet with Onions and Peppers, 4–5
Just Like Takeout Sweet-and-Sour Chicken, 72–73★
My Dad's Trim Chicken Enchiladas, 67★
Pork Lo Mein, Hold the Grease, 92–93
quick meals with, 177–78
Rainbow Macaroni Salad with Tuna, 60

Sesame Chicken Hold the Deep-Fried
Breading, 74–75
Spicy Sloppy Joes with Carrot and
Red Bell Pepper, 94–95
Stuffed Peppers Cooked in Pepperoni-
Flavored Tomato Sauce, 58–59
Supermoist Turkey Burgers, 82–83
Berries
adding to muffin recipe, 18
blueberries, health benefits, 20
Blueberry Cobbler with Yogurt
Topping, 134–35
Chocolate-Covered Pretzels and
Fruit, 155
Frozen Fruit Skewers, 156
Italian Cheesecake, 143
Peanut Butter Spread and Jelly on
Toast, 20
Ricotta Strawberry Shortcake Parfait,
154
Biscuits
Buttermilk Biscuits, 125
Black beans
Creamy Mexican Bean Dip with
Whole Grain Tortilla Chips, 41
Garlicky Black Bean Soup, 30–31
Nachos Grande with Pickled Jalapeño
Salsa, 42–43
Southwestern Frittata with Spicy
Corn Salsa, 8–9★
Tantalizing Turkey Tacos with Star
Anise, 84–85
Blueberries
Blueberry Cobbler with Yogurt
Topping, 134–35
health benefits, 20
Peanut Butter Spread and Jelly on
Toast, 20
Blue cheese
adding to salad dressing, 176
Stuffed Mushrooms with Blue
Cheese, 107
Twice-Baked Potatoes with Filling So
Rich No One Will Know It's Low
Fat, 104
Breads. See also Pita bread; Tortillas
Banana Bread, 150–51
Buttermilk Biscuits, 125
French Onion Soup with Cheesy
Whole Wheat Croutons, 28–29★
French Toast with Orange
Marmalade, 16
Lemony Yogurt Muffins, 18–19
Party Dip Served with Whole Wheat
Pita, 45
Peanut Butter Spread and Jelly on
Toast, 20
whole-wheat bread crumbs,
preparing, 89

Whole Wheat Garlic Bread,
126–27
Zucchini Bread for Breakfast, Too,
152–53
Breakfast
Apple Butter, 21
Bacon, Egg, and Cheese Sandwich, 3
Bacon Sausage Omelet with Onions
and Peppers, 4–5
Baked Eggs and Ham, 6
Blender Pancakes with Sweet
Cinnamon Bananas, 10–11
Chocolate Breakfast Shake, 22
Essential Smoothie, 23
French Toast with Orange
Marmalade, 16
Homemade Granola Bars, 17
importance of, 15
Lemony Yogurt Muffins, 18–19
Maple Apple Waffles, 14–15
My Granny's Cinnamon Coffee Cake
the Skinny Way, 140–41
Peanut Butter Spread and Jelly on
Toast, 20
Scrambled Eggs to Go, 7
Southwestern Frittata with Spicy
Corn Salsa, 8–9★
Zucchini Bread for Breakfast, Too,
152–53
Zucchini Pancakes with Walnuts and
Spice, 12–13
Broccoli
adding to meatballs, 185
Broccoli Bacon Salad, 113
Chicken Marsala with Mushrooms
and Broccoli, 80–81
"Cream" of Broccoli Soup with
Cheddar, 36
Just Like Takeout Sweet-and-Sour
Chicken, 72–73★
Nachos Grande with Pickled Jalapeño
Salsa, 42–43
quick meals with, 177–78
Rainbow Macaroni Salad with Tuna,
60
Stir-Fried Garlic Broccoli, 123
Tender Beef Stroganoff, 98–99
Brownies
Slender Blondie Brownies with
Walnuts, Chocolate Chips, and
Prunes, 146–47★
Burgers
adding chopped mushrooms to, 184
Supermoist Turkey Burgers, 82–83
Buttermilk
Banana Bread, 150–51
Buttermilk Biscuits, 125
Buttermilk Yogurt Dressing, 117
Cherry Sherbet, 158

Cabbage
"Mayonnaise Is Not Your Enemy"
Coleslaw, 112
Pigs in a Blanket, 90–91
Cakes
Carrot Cake with Applesauce and
Carrot Juice, 136–37
Chocolate Angel Food Cupcakes with
Angelic Icing, 138–39
My Granny's Cinnamon Coffee Cake
the Skinny Way, 140–41
Sinful Chocolate Cake Made with
Raisins and Bittersweet Morsels,
142
Calories, xxvii
Carbohydrates, xxi–xxii
Carrot juice
Carrot Cake with Applesauce and
Carrot Juice, 136–37
Chocolate Pudding Pops, 157
Essential Smoothie, 23
Whole Wheat Garlic Bread, 126–27
Carrots. See also Carrot juice
Carrot Cake with Applesauce and
Carrot Juice, 136–37
Carrot Ginger Dressing, 118
grated, adding to frozen treats, 158
grated, adding to tomato sauce, 184
Honey-Roasted Baby Carrots with
Raisins, 121
"Mayonnaise Is Not Your Enemy"
Coleslaw, 112
Meatball Sandwiches, 88–89★
Party Dip Served with Whole Wheat
Pita, 45
Spicy Sloppy Joes with Carrot and
Red Bell Pepper, 94–95
Zucchini Pancakes with Walnuts and
Spice, 12–13
Catfish
Cajun Catfish in Cornmeal Breading,
61
Cauliflower
Broccoli Bacon Salad, 113
Chicken "No Pot Belly" Pie, 70–71
Mac and Cheese with Shredded
Chicken and Cauliflower,
52–53★
Celery
Hot "Wings" with Spicy Sauce, 44
Party Dip Served with Whole Wheat
Pita, 45
Cheddar cheese
"Cream" of Broccoli Soup with
Cheddar, 36
Cheese
adding to salad dressing, 176
Bacon, Egg, and Cheese Sandwich, 3
Baked Eggs and Ham, 6

Cheese (cont.)
   Carrot Cake with Applesauce and
      Carrot Juice, 136–37
   "Cream" of Broccoli Soup with
      Cheddar, 36
   Creamy Mexican Bean Dip with
      Whole Grain Tortilla Chips, 41
   Cut the Fat, Keep the Creamy Pasta
      Carbonara, 51
   French Onion Soup with Cheesy
      Whole Wheat Croutons, 28–29★
   French Tuna Salad, 62–63
   Good Lookin' Grilled Cheese, 57
   Italian Cheesecake, 143
   Light Lasagna Made with Turkey and
      Veggies, 54–55★
   Mac and Cheese with Shredded
      Chicken and Cauliflower, 52–53★
   Meatball Sandwiches, 88–89★
   My Dad's Trim Chicken Enchiladas,
      67★
   Nachos Grande with Pickled Jalapeño
      Salsa, 42–43
   ricotta, adding to shakes or dessert,
      184
   Ricotta Strawberry Shortcake Parfait,
      154
   Scalloped Potatoes with Ham, 105–6
   Southwestern Frittata with Spicy
      Corn Salsa, 8–9★
   Stuffed Chicken Parmesan, 66
   Stuffed Mushrooms with Blue
      Cheese, 107
   Stuffed Shells That Won't Leave You
      Feeling Stuffed, 56★
   Tiramisu Parfaits, 144–45★
   Twice-Baked Potatoes with Filling So
      Rich No One Will Know It's Low
      Fat, 104
Cheesecake
   Italian Cheesecake, 143
Cherries
   Cherry Sherbet, 158
Chicken
   Bacon Spinach Salad, 116
   Baked "Deep Fried" Chicken with
      Crunchy Double Whole Grain
      Breading, 68–69
   Chicken and Rice Hot Pot, 76–77
   Chicken Marsala with Mushrooms
      and Broccoli, 80–81
   Chicken "No Pot Belly" Pie, 70–71
   Chicken Paprikash, Creamy but Light
      Chicken Stew, 78–79
   cooking tips, 66, 81, 82
   flavoring, with herbs and spices, 82
   Hot "Wings" with Spicy Sauce, 44
   Just Like Takeout Sweet-and-Sour
      Chicken, 72–73★
   Mac and Cheese with Shredded

   Chicken and Cauliflower, 52–53★
   My Dad's Trim Chicken Enchiladas,
      67★
   Sesame Chicken Hold the Deep-Fried
      Breading, 74–75
   Stuffed Chicken Parmesan, 66
   Ten-Minute Chicken Noodle Soup, 38
Chicken sausages
   Bacon Sausage Omelet with Onions
      and Peppers, 4–5
   quick meal idea with, 178
Chile peppers
   Alarmingly Good Low-Fat Chili, 34–35
   Garlicky Black Bean Soup, 30–31
   Nachos Grande with Pickled Jalapeño
      Salsa, 42–43
   Pigs in a Blanket, 90–91
   Rainbow Macaroni Salad with Tuna,
      60
   Shrimp and Corn Fritters, 110–11
   Southwestern Frittata with Spicy
      Corn Salsa, 8–9★
Chili
   adding vegetables to, 35
   Alarmingly Good Low-Fat Chili, 34–35
Chocolate
   Chocolate Angel Food Cupcakes with
      Angelic Icing, 138–39
   Chocolate Breakfast Shake, 22
   Chocolate-Covered Pretzels and
      Fruit, 155
   Chocolate Pudding Pops, 157
   Hot Fudge Sundae with Vanilla Bean
      Frozen Yogurt, 161
   Sinful Chocolate Cake Made with
      Raisins and Bittersweet Morsels,
      142
   Slender Blondie Brownies with
      Walnuts, Chocolate Chips, and
      Prunes, 146–47★
   Tiramisu Parfaits, 144–45★
Chowder
   Shrimp and Corn Chowder, 37★
Cilantro
   Garlicky Black Bean Soup, 30–31
   Nachos Grande with Pickled Jalapeño
      Salsa, 42–43
   Southwestern Frittata with Spicy
      Corn Salsa, 8–9★
Cinnamon
   Banana Bread, 150–51
   My Granny's Cinnamon Coffee Cake
      the Skinny Way, 140–41
Coconut
   Butternut Squash Soup with Coconut
      Milk, 27
   Frozen Coconut Yogurt, 159★
   Frozen Fruit Skewers, 156
Coffee
   Tiramisu Parfaits, 144–45★

Coffee cake
   My Granny's Cinnamon Coffee Cake
      the Skinny Way, 140–41
Collard greens
   Four Food Groups Minestrone, 32–33
   Pork Lo Mein, Hold the Grease, 92–93
Cookies and bars
   Homemade Granola Bars, 17
   Slender Blondie Brownies with
      Walnuts, Chocolate Chips, and
      Prunes, 146–47★
Corn
   Shrimp and Corn Chowder, 37★
   Shrimp and Corn Fritters, 110–11
   Southwestern Frittata with Spicy
      Corn Salsa, 8–9★
Cottage cheese
   Tiramisu Parfaits, 144–45★
Cranberries, adding to muffin recipe, 18
Cream cheese
   Carrot Cake with Applesauce and
      Carrot Juice, 136–37
Cucumbers
   Cucumber Salad with Sour Cream
      and Fresh Dill, 115
Cupcakes
   Chocolate Angel Food Cupcakes with
      Angelic Icing, 138–39

Dairy products. See also specific dairy
   products
   daily recommended servings, xxviii
   low-fat, cooking with, 78
Dates
   Bacon-Wrapped Dates, 40
Desserts
   Apple Strudel with Walnut Crumble
      Topping, 148–49
   Banana Bread, 150–51
   Banana Cream Pie, 132–33★
   Blueberry Cobbler with Yogurt
      Topping, 134–35
   Carrot Cake with Applesauce and
      Carrot Juice, 136–37
   Cherry Sherbet, 158
   Chocolate Angel Food Cupcakes with
      Angelic Icing, 138–39
   Chocolate-Covered Pretzels and
      Fruit, 155
   Chocolate Pudding Pops, 157
   Crustless Apple Pie, 131
   Frozen Coconut Yogurt, 159★
   Frozen Fruit Skewers, 156
   Hot Fudge Sundae with Vanilla Bean
      Frozen Yogurt, 161
   Italian Cheesecake, 143
   My Granny's Cinnamon Coffee Cake
      the Skinny Way, 140–41

Ricotta Strawberry Shortcake Parfait, 154

Sinful Chocolate Cake Made with Raisins and Bittersweet Morsels, 142

Slender Blondie Brownies with Walnuts, Chocolate Chips, and Prunes, 146–47★

Tiramisu Parfaits, 144–45★

Vanilla Bean "Ice Cream," 160

Zucchini Bread for Breakfast, Too, 152–53

Diets and dieting, xix, xxi, 47

Diet shakes, store-bought, about, 22

Dinner. See Main dishes; Side dishes

Dips and spreads

Apple Butter, 21

Creamy Mexican Bean Dip with Whole Grain Tortilla Chips, 41

healthy, preparing, 41

Party Dip Served with Whole Wheat Pita, 45

Peanut Butter Spread and Jelly on Toast, 20

Dressings. See Salad dressings

Drinks

Chocolate Breakfast Shake, 22

Essential Smoothie, 23

store-bought diet shakes, about, 22

Eggs

Bacon, Egg, and Cheese Sandwich, 3

Bacon Sausage Omelet with Onions and Peppers, 4–5

Bacon Spinach Salad, 116

Baked Eggs and Ham, 6

Cut the Fat, Keep the Creamy Pasta Carbonara, 51

French Tuna Salad, 62–63

Garlicky Black Bean Soup, 30–31

Rainbow Macaroni Salad with Tuna, 60

Scrambled Eggs to Go, 7

Southwestern Frittata with Spicy Corn Salsa, 8–9★

whole, substitute for, 4

Enchiladas

My Dad's Trim Chicken Enchiladas, 67★

Endives

Bacon-Wrapped Dates, 40

Fats, dietary

cooking oils, note about, 93

daily recommended intake, xx–xxi

importance of, xxiii

omega-3 fatty acids, xxi

saturated fat, 3

saturated fats, xxi

vitamin absorption and, 175

Fennel

"Mayonnaise Is Not Your Enemy" Coleslaw, 112

Fiber, xxii, xxiii

Fish

Cajun Catfish in Cornmeal Breading, 61

cooking tip, 66

French Tuna Salad, 62–63

Mock Crab Cakes with Zucchini and Tuna, 64

omega-3 fatty acids in, xxi

Rainbow Macaroni Salad with Tuna, 60

Seven-Minute Salmon, 65

Flaxseed

adding to desserts, 135

adding to frozen treats, 158

Alarmingly Good Low-Fat Chili, 34–35

Banana Cream Pie, 132–33★

Blueberry Cobbler with Yogurt Topping, 134–35

Chocolate-Covered Pretzels and Fruit, 155

Essential Smoothie, 23

Frozen Coconut Yogurt, 159★

ground, cooking with, 23

health benefits, 23

Homemade Granola Bars, 17

Maple Apple Waffles, 14–15

omega-3 fatty acids in, xxi

Party Dip Served with Whole Wheat Pita, 45

Party Mix with Spiced Nuts and Whole Grain Cereal, 46–47

Peanut Butter Spread and Jelly on Toast, 20

storing, 23

Whole Wheat Garlic Bread, 126–27

Zucchini Pancakes with Walnuts and Spice, 12–13

Flour, white whole-wheat, about, 146

French-style dishes

Bacon Sausage Omelet with Onions and Peppers, 4–5

French Onion Soup with Cheesy Whole Wheat Croutons, 28–29★

French Tuna Salad, 62–63

Frittatas

Southwestern Frittata with Spicy Corn Salsa, 8–9★

Fritters

Shrimp and Corn Fritters, 110–11

Fruits. See also specific fruits

adding to muffin recipe, 18

Chocolate-Covered Pretzels and Fruit, 155

daily recommended servings, xxvii

Frozen Fruit Skewers, 156

as oil substitute in desserts, 137

Garlic

Garlicky Black Bean Soup, 30–31

Simple Sautéed Spinach with Garlic and Chile Flakes, 122

Stir-Fried Garlic Broccoli, 123

Whole Wheat Garlic Bread, 126–27

Ginger

Carrot Ginger Dressing, 118

Sesame Chicken Hold the Deep-Fried Breading, 74–75

Seven-Minute Salmon, 65

Shrimp and Corn Fritters, 110–11

Stir-Fried Garlic Broccoli, 123

Grains. See also Oats; Quinoa; Rice

adding to baked goods, 152

adding to pancake batter, 11, 152

adding to waffle batter, 152

daily recommended servings, xxviii

Party Mix with Spiced Nuts and Whole Grain Cereal, 46–47

wheat germ, adding to muffin recipe, 18

whole, health benefits from, xxi–xxii

whole, increasing intake of, xxiii

Grapes

Frozen Fruit Skewers, 156

Poolside Soup, 39

Green beans

French Tuna Salad, 62–63

Green Beans with Almonds and Lemon Pepper Croutons, 120

Three Bean Salad, 114

Greens. See also Spinach

best, for salads, 176

Four Food Groups Minestrone, 32–33

French Tuna Salad, 62–63

mixed baby greens, buying, 176

Pork Lo Mein, Hold the Grease, 92–93

romaine lettuce, health benefits, 85

Ham

Baked Eggs and Ham, 6

Scalloped Potatoes with Ham, 105–6

Heart disease, xxi

Herbs. See also Basil; Cilantro; Mint

fresh, cooking with, 6

Horseradish

Party Dip Served with Whole Wheat Pita, 45

Hunger pangs, preventing, 77

Ice cream
Vanilla Bean "Ice Cream," 160
Italian-style dishes
Baked Meatballs with Zesty Marinara,
86–87
Chicken Marsala with Mushrooms
and Broccoli, 80–81
Cut the Fat, Keep the Creamy Pasta
Carbonara, 51
Four Food Groups Minestrone, 32–33
Italian Cheesecake, 143
Light Lasagna Made with Turkey and
Veggies, 54–55★
Southwestern Frittata with Spicy
Corn Salsa, 8–9★
Stuffed Chicken Parmesan, 66
Stuffed Peppers Cooked in Pepperoni-
Flavored Tomato Sauce, 58–59
Stuffed Shells That Won't Leave You
Feeling Stuffed, 56★
Tiramisu Parfaits, 144–45★

Kiwifruit
Poolside Soup, 39

Lasagna
Light Lasagna Made with Turkey and
Veggies, 54–55★
Leftovers, ideas for, 180–83
Lemons
Lemony Yogurt Muffins, 18–19
as salad dressing, 176
Lettuce
choosing, for salads, 176
romaine, health benefits, 85, 176
Limes
Seven-Minute Salmon, 65
Shrimp and Corn Fritters, 110–11
Lunch
Alarmingly Good Low-Fat Chili,
34–35
Bacon Spinach Salad, 116
Broccoli Bacon Salad, 113
Butternut Squash Soup with Coconut
Milk, 27
"Cream" of Broccoli Soup with
Cheddar, 36
Cucumber Salad with Sour Cream
and Fresh Dill, 115
Four Food Groups Minestrone, 32–33
French Onion Soup with Cheesy
Whole Wheat Croutons, 28–29★
French Tuna Salad, 62–63
Garlicky Black Bean Soup, 30–31

Good Lookin' Grilled Cheese, 57
Light Lasagna Made with Turkey and
Veggies, 54–55★
Mac and Cheese with Shredded
Chicken and Cauliflower, 52–53★
"Mayonnaise Is Not Your Enemy"
Coleslaw, 112
Meatball Sandwiches, 88–89★
Mock Crab Cakes with Zucchini and
Tuna, 64
Poolside Soup, 39
Rainbow Macaroni Salad with Tuna,
60
Shrimp and Corn Chowder, 37★
Spicy Sloppy Joes with Carrot and
Red Bell Pepper, 94–95
Stuffed Shells That Won't Leave You
Feeling Stuffed, 56★
Supermoist Turkey Burgers, 82–83
Ten-Minute Chicken Noodle Soup,
38
Three Bean Salad, 114

Main dishes
Alarmingly Good Low-Fat Chili,
34–35
Baked "Deep Fried" Chicken with
Crunchy Double Whole Grain
Breading, 68–69
Baked Meatballs with Zesty Marinara,
86–87
Cajun Catfish in Cornmeal Breading,
61
Chicken and Rice Hot Pot, 76–77
Chicken Marsala with Mushrooms
and Broccoli, 80–81
Chicken "No Pot Belly" Pie, 70–71
Chicken Paprikash, Creamy but Light
Chicken Stew, 78–79
Cut the Fat, Keep the Creamy Pasta
Carbonara, 51
Four Food Groups Minestrone, 32–33
French Tuna Salad, 62–63
Garlicky Black Bean Soup, 30–31
Good Lookin' Grilled Cheese, 57
Just Like Takeout Sweet-and-Sour
Chicken, 72–73★
Light Lasagna Made with Turkey and
Veggies, 54–55★
Mac and Cheese with Shredded
Chicken and Cauliflower, 52–53★
Meatball Sandwiches, 88–89★
Mock Crab Cakes with Zucchini and
Tuna, 6
My Dad's Trim Chicken Enchiladas,
67★
Pigs in a Blanket, 90–91

Pork Lo Mein, Hold the Grease,
92–93
Rainbow Macaroni Salad with Tuna,
60
Sesame Chicken Hold the Deep-Fried
Breading, 74–75
Seven-Minute Salmon, 65
Spicy Sloppy Joes with Carrot and
Red Bell Pepper, 94–95
Steak and Potatoes, 96–97★
Stuffed Chicken Parmesan, 66
Stuffed Peppers Cooked in Pepperoni-
Flavored Tomato Sauce, 58–59
Stuffed Shells That Won't Leave You
Feeling Stuffed, 56★
Supermoist Turkey Burgers, 82–83
Tantalizing Turkey Tacos with Star
Anise, 84–85
Tender Beef Stroganoff, 98–99
Mandolines, Japanese, 105
Mangoes
Frozen Fruit Skewers, 156
Maple syrup
Maple Apple Waffles, 14–15
Meatballs
adding chopped broccoli to, 185
Baked Meatballs with Zesty Marinara,
86–87
Meatball Sandwiches, 88–89★
Microplane slicers, 16
Milk, adding to soups, 184
Mint
Poolside Soup, 39
Rainbow Macaroni Salad with Tuna,
60
Mozzarella cheese
Bacon, Egg, and Cheese Sandwich, 3
Baked Eggs and Ham, 6
Creamy Mexican Bean Dip with
Whole Grain Tortilla Chips, 41
French Onion Soup with Cheesy
Whole Wheat Croutons, 28–29★
French Tuna Salad, 62–63
Good Lookin' Grilled Cheese, 57
Light Lasagna Made with Turkey and
Veggies, 54–55★
Mac and Cheese with Shredded
Chicken and Cauliflower,
52–53★
Meatball Sandwiches, 88–89★
My Dad's Trim Chicken Enchiladas,
67★
Nachos Grande with Pickled Jalapeño
Salsa, 42–43
Southwestern Frittata with Spicy
Corn Salsa, 8–9★
Stuffed Chicken Parmesan, 66
Stuffed Shells That Won't Leave You
Feeling Stuffed, 56★

Muffins
    add-ins for, 18
    Lemony Yogurt Muffins, 18–19
Mushrooms
    adding to turkey burgers, 184
    Bacon Spinach Salad, 116
    Baked Eggs and Ham, 6
    Chicken Marsala with Mushrooms
        and Broccoli, 80–81
    My Dad's Trim Chicken Enchiladas,
        67★
    Pork Lo Mein, Hold the Grease,
        92–93
    quick meals with, 177
    Stuffed Mushrooms with Blue
        Cheese, 107
    Supermoist Turkey Burgers, 82–83
    Tender Beef Stroganoff, 98–99

Nachos
    Nachos Grande with Pickled Jalapeño
        Salsa, 42–43
Noodles
    Pork Lo Mein, Hold the Grease, 92–93
    Ten-Minute Chicken Noodle Soup,
        38
Nutrition labels, xxiii–xxiv, 175, 178
Nuts. See also Almonds; Walnuts
    Frozen Fruit Skewers, 156
    Party Mix with Spiced Nuts and
        Whole Grain Cereal, 46–47

Oats
    Blueberry Cobbler with Yogurt
        Topping, 134–35
    Crustless Apple Pie, 131
    Homemade Granola Bars, 17
Olives
    adding to salad dressing, 176
    Chicken and Rice Hot Pot, 76–77
    Creamy Mexican Bean Dip with
        Whole Grain Tortilla Chips, 41
    French Tuna Salad, 62–63
Omega-3 fatty acids, xxi, 23
Omelets
    Bacon Sausage Omelet with Onions
        and Peppers, 4–5
Onions
    French Onion Soup with Cheesy
        Whole Wheat Croutons, 28–29★
Orange marmalade
    French Toast with Orange
        Marmalade, 16
    Just Like Takeout Sweet-and-Sour
        Chicken, 72–73★

Oranges
    Chocolate-Covered Pretzels and
        Fruit, 155
    Essential Smoothie, 23
    French Toast with Orange
        Marmalade, 16
    Just Like Takeout Sweet-and-Sour
        Chicken, 72–73★
    Pork Lo Mein, Hold the Grease,
        92–93

Pancakes
    adding whole grains to, 11, 152
    Blender Pancakes with Sweet
        Cinnamon Bananas, 10–11
    Zucchini Pancakes with Walnuts and
        Spice, 12–13
Parfaits
    Ricotta Strawberry Shortcake Parfait,
        154
    Tiramisu Parfaits, 144–45★
Parmesan cheese
    Cut the Fat, Keep the Creamy Pasta
        Carbonara, 51
    Scalloped Potatoes with Ham, 105–6
    Stuffed Shells That Won't Leave You
        Feeling Stuffed, 56★
Pasta. See also Noodles
    Cut the Fat, Keep the Creamy Pasta
        Carbonara, 51
    Four Food Groups Minestrone, 32–33
    Light Lasagna Made with Turkey and
        Veggies, 54–55★
    Mac and Cheese with Shredded
        Chicken and Cauliflower, 52–53★
    Rainbow Macaroni Salad with Tuna,
        60
    Stuffed Shells That Won't Leave You
        Feeling Stuffed, 56★
Peaches
    Hot Fudge Sundae with Vanilla Bean
        Frozen Yogurt, 161
    as oil substitute in desserts, 137
Peanut butter
    Homemade Granola Bars, 17
    Peanut Butter Spread and Jelly on
        Toast, 20
    Pork Lo Mein, Hold the Grease, 92–93
    Seven-Minute Salmon, 65
Pears
    My Granny's Cinnamon Coffee Cake
        the Skinny Way, 140–41
    as oil substitute in desserts, 137
Pecans
    Frozen Fruit Skewers, 156
    Party Mix with Spiced Nuts and
        Whole Grain Cereal, 46–47

Pepperoni
    Stuffed Peppers Cooked in Pepperoni-
        Flavored Tomato Sauce, 58–59
Peppers. See Bell peppers; Chile peppers
Phyllo dough
    about, 71
    Apple Strudel with Walnut Crumble
        Topping, 148–49
    Chicken "No Pot Belly" Pie, 70–71
Pies
    Banana Cream Pie, 132–33★
    Crustless Apple Pie, 131
Pineapple
    Just Like Takeout Sweet-and-Sour
        Chicken, 72–73★
    Zucchini Bread for Breakfast, Too,
        152–53
Pita bread
    Baked Eggs and Ham, 6
    Scrambled Eggs to Go, 7
Pork
    Baked Eggs and Ham, 6
    Pork Lo Mein, Hold the Grease,
        92–93
    Scalloped Potatoes with Ham, 105–6
    Stuffed Peppers Cooked in Pepperoni-
        Flavored Tomato Sauce, 58–59
Portion sizes, xxii–xxiii, xxvii–xxviii,
    31, 63
Potatoes
    Baked Steak House Fries, 103★
    "Cream" of Broccoli Soup with
        Cheddar, 36
    French Tuna Salad, 62–63
    mashed, adding to soups, 27
    Scalloped Potatoes with Ham, 105–6
    Shrimp and Corn Chowder, 37★
    Steak and Potatoes, 96–97★
    Twice-Baked Potatoes with Filling So
        Rich No One Will Know It's Low
        Fat, 104
Pot pies
    Chicken "No Pot Belly" Pie, 70–71
Pretzels
    Chocolate-Covered Pretzels and
        Fruit, 155
    Party Mix with Spiced Nuts and
        Whole Grain Cereal, 46–47
Protein
    adding to salads, 177
    daily recommended servings, xxviii
    hunger-busting effects of, 77
Prunes
    adding to muffin recipe, 18
    Apple Strudel with Walnut Crumble
        Topping, 148–49
    Carrot Cake with Applesauce and
        Carrot Juice, 136–37
    Homemade Granola Bars, 17

Prunes (cont.)
  Slender Blondie Brownies with
    Walnuts, Chocolate Chips, and
    Prunes, 146–47★
Pumpkin seeds
  Essential Smoothie, 23
  Homemade Granola Bars, 17
  Party Mix with Spiced Nuts and
    Whole Grain Cereal, 46–47

Quesadillas, for quick meals, 178
Quinoa
  French Tuna Salad, 62–63
  Zucchini Bread for Breakfast, Too,
    152–53

Raisins
  Apple Strudel with Walnut Crumble
    Topping, 148–49
  Broccoli Bacon Salad, 113
  Honey-Roasted Baby Carrots with
    Raisins, 121
  Sinful Chocolate Cake Made with
    Raisins and Bittersweet Morsels,
    142
  Zucchini Bread for Breakfast, Too,
    152–53
Raspberries
  Frozen Fruit Skewers, 156
Recipe index by category
  brunch, 170–71
  celiac-safe, 173–74
  easy to cook with kids, 168
  finger food for football games and
    parties, 170
  holidays, 169–70
  kid friendly, 167–68
  one-pot meals or desserts for potlucks,
    168
  restaurant favorites, 171
  romantic dinner for two, 172–73
  school or work lunch, 167
  super fast week night, 172
  tapas or cocktail party, 171–72
  work out before and after, 170
Recipes
  adding fridge odds and ends to,
    184–85
  leftovers from, ideas for, 180–83
  shopping list for, 163–65
Rice
  brown, adding to recipes, 185
  Chicken and Rice Hot Pot, 76–77
  Chicken Paprikash, Creamy but Light
    Chicken Stew, 78–79

Just Like Takeout Sweet-and-Sour
    Chicken, 72–73★
  Pigs in a Blanket, 90–91
  Sesame Chicken Hold the Deep-Fried
    Breading, 74–75
  Stuffed Peppers Cooked in Pepperoni-
    Flavored Tomato Sauce, 58–59
  Tender Beef Stroganoff, 98–99
Ricotta cheese
  adding to shakes or dessert, 184
  Italian Cheesecake, 143
  Light Lasagna Made with Turkey and
    Veggies, 54–55★
  My Dad's Trim Chicken Enchiladas,
    67★
  Ricotta Strawberry Shortcake Parfait,
    154
  Stuffed Shells That Won't Leave You
    Feeling Stuffed, 56★

Salad dressings
  Almond Dressing, 119
  Buttermilk Yogurt Dressing, 117
  Carrot Ginger Dressing, 118
  homemade, benefits of, 117
  homemade, preparing, 175–76
  store-bought, reading nutritional
    labels on, 175
Salads
  Bacon Spinach Salad, 116
  Broccoli Bacon Salad, 113
  Cucumber Salad with Sour Cream
    and Fresh Dill, 115
  French Tuna Salad, 62–63
  greens for, 176
  main dish, preparing, 175–77
  "Mayonnaise Is Not Your Enemy"
    Coleslaw, 112
  Rainbow Macaroni Salad with Tuna,
    60
  Three Bean Salad, 114
Salmon
  Seven-Minute Salmon, 65
Salsa
  Pickled Jalapeño Salsa, 42–43
  as salad dressing, 176
Sandwiches and burgers
  Bacon, Egg, and Cheese Sandwich, 3
  Good Lookin' Grilled Cheese, 57
  Meatball Sandwiches, 88–89★
  Scrambled Eggs to Go, 7
  Spicy Sloppy Joes with Carrot and
    Red Bell Pepper, 94–95
  Supermoist Turkey Burgers, 82–83
Saturated fat, xxi, 3
Sauces
  dry, remedy for, 51

healthy, preparing, 41
  Sweet Chile Sauce, 110–11
Sausages, chicken
  Bacon Sausage Omelet with Onions
    and Peppers, 4–5
  quick meal idea with, 178
Sesame seeds
  Homemade Granola Bars, 17
  Sesame Chicken Hold the Deep-Fried
    Breading, 74–75
Shellfish
  shrimp, quick meal idea with, 177–78
  Shrimp and Corn Chowder, 37★
  Shrimp and Corn Fritters, 110–11
Sherbet
  Cherry Sherbet, 158
Shrimp
  quick meals with, 177–78
  Shrimp and Corn Chowder, 37★
  Shrimp and Corn Fritters, 110–11
Side dishes
  Bacon Spinach Salad, 116
  Baked Steak House Fries, 103★
  Breaded Zucchini with Marinara
    Dipping Sauce, 108–9★
  Broccoli Bacon Salad, 113
  Buttermilk Biscuits, 125
  Cucumber Salad with Sour Cream
    and Fresh Dill, 115
  Green Beans with Almonds and
    Lemon Pepper Croutons, 120
  Honey-Roasted Baby Carrots with
    Raisins, 121
  "Mayonnaise Is Not Your Enemy"
    Coleslaw, 112
  Scalloped Potatoes with Ham, 105–6
  Shrimp and Corn Fritters, 110–11
  Simple Sautéed Spinach with Garlic
    and Chile Flakes, 122
  Stir-Fried Garlic Broccoli, 123
  Stuffed Mushrooms with Blue
    Cheese, 107
  Three Bean Salad, 114
  Twice-Baked Potatoes with Filling So
    Rich No One Will Know It's Low
    Fat, 104
  Warm Creamed Spinach Minus the
    Heavy Cream, 124
  Whole Wheat Garlic Bread, 126–27
Skinny Chef resources
  free handy reference chart, 187
  online audio lesson, 187
  online cooking videos, 186
  online shopping list, 186
  quick start booklet, 187
  Skinny Shopping List, 163–65
  weekly expert tips, 187
Skinny Secrets
  adding cooked grains to waffles, 152

adding flaxseed to desserts, 135
adding hunger-busting protein to meals, 77
adding vegetables to recipes, 13, 35, 57
adding vinegar to baked goods, 150
adding whole grains to pancakes, 11, 152
avoiding dieting fads, xxi
avoiding fat-laden take-out food, 73, 97
avoiding store-bought diet shakes, 22
baking with phyllo dough, 71
baking with white whole wheat flour, 146
buying quality ingredients, 43
choosing locally grown food, 149
choosing quick-cooking foods, 65
cooking chicken over high heat, 81
cooking for children, 87
cooking low-fat protein, 66, 82
cooking with canned tomatoes, 90
cooking with fresh herbs, 6
cooking with low-fat dairy products, 78
cooking with savory spices and sauces, 75
cooking with spinach, 122, 124
cooking with Sriracha, 111
cooking with turkey bacon, 3
cutting back on oil, 93
drinking more water, xxiv–xxv
eating blueberries, 20
eating breakfast, 15
eating flaxseed, 23
eating more vegetables, xx
eating whole grains, xxi–xxii
ending mindless eating, 55
fixing bad eating habits, 29
fixing dry sauces or casseroles, 51
homemade frozen treats, 158
homemade tomato sauce, 89
homemade whole-wheat bread crumbs, 89
learning about fats, xx–xxi
learning to enjoy food preparation, 55
making favorite recipes healthier, 47, 52
making lighter versions of bar food, 44
making weeknight meals special, 56
making your own salad dressing, 117
preparing creamless creamy soups, 27
preparing "faux" fried foods, 69
preparing healthy dips and sauces, 41
preserving rich flavors in recipes, 40
reading nutrition labels, xxiii–xxiv

readjusting portion sizes, xxii–xxiii, 31, 63
seasoning with cayenne or chile flakes, 61
sharing a healthy brunch, 9
slicing beef, 99
stocking healthy pantry items, 109
substituting egg whites for yolks, 4
switching to healthier ingredients, 85
using mandoline, 105
using oil substitutes in baked goods, 137
using zester or microplane, 16
Slaws
    "Mayonnaise Is Not Your Enemy" Coleslaw, 112
Snacks, healthy, suggestions for, 178–79
Soda, xxiv
Soups. See also Stews
    adding vegetables to, 35
    Butternut Squash Soup with Coconut Milk, 27
    "Cream" of Broccoli Soup with Cheddar, 36
    Four Food Groups Minestrone, 32–33
    French Onion Soup with Cheesy Whole Wheat Croutons, 28–29★
    Garlicky Black Bean Soup, 30–31
    Poolside Soup, 39
    preparing creamless creamy soups, 27
    Shrimp and Corn Chowder, 37★
    Ten-Minute Chicken Noodle Soup, 38
Southwestern-style dishes
    Alarmingly Good Low-Fat Chili, 34–35
    Creamy Mexican Bean Dip with Whole Grain Tortilla Chips, 41
    Garlicky Black Bean Soup, 30–31
    My Dad's Trim Chicken Enchiladas, 67★
    Nachos Grande with Pickled Jalapeño Salsa, 42–43
    Southwestern Frittata with Spicy Corn Salsa, 8–9★
    Tantalizing Turkey Tacos with Star Anise, 84–85
Spinach
    adding to frozen treats, 158
    Bacon Spinach Salad, 116
    Baked Meatballs with Zesty Marinara, 86–87
    "Cream" of Broccoli Soup with Cheddar, 36
    Creamy Mexican Bean Dip with Whole Grain Tortilla Chips, 41
    health benefits, 124, 176
    Mock Crab Cakes with Zucchini and Tuna, 64

Nachos Grande with Pickled Jalapeño Salsa, 42–43
Party Dip Served with Whole Wheat Pita, 45
quick cooking times, 122, 124
Scrambled Eggs to Go, 7
Sesame Chicken Hold the Deep-Fried Breading, 74–75
Simple Sautéed Spinach with Garlic and Chile Flakes, 122
Southwestern Frittata with Spicy Corn Salsa, 8–9★
Stuffed Shells That Won't Leave You Feeling Stuffed, 56★
Supermoist Turkey Burgers, 82–83
Warm Creamed Spinach Minus the Heavy Cream, 124
Squash
    Breaded Zucchini with Marinara Dipping Sauce, 108–9★
    Butternut Squash Soup with Coconut Milk, 27
    Meatball Sandwiches, 88–89★
    Mock Crab Cakes with Zucchini and Tuna, 64
    Zucchini Bread for Breakfast, Too, 152–53
    Zucchini Pancakes with Walnuts and Spice, 12–13
Sriracha
    about, 111
    Sesame Chicken Hold the Deep-Fried Breading, 74–75
    Shrimp and Corn Fritters, 110–11
Star anise
    Apple Butter, 21
    Tantalizing Turkey Tacos with Star Anise, 84–85
Stews
    Alarmingly Good Low-Fat Chili, 34–35
    Chicken and Rice Hot Pot, 76–77
    Chicken Paprikash, Creamy but Light Chicken Stew, 78–79
Strawberries
    Chocolate-Covered Pretzels and Fruit, 155
    Italian Cheesecake, 143
    Ricotta Strawberry Shortcake Parfait, 154
Strudel
    Apple Strudel with Walnut Crumble Topping, 148–49
Sweet potatoes
    mashed, adding to soups, 27
    Scalloped Potatoes with Ham, 105–6
Swiss cheese
    Good Lookin' Grilled Cheese, 57
    Scalloped Potatoes with Ham, 105–6

Tacos
 Tantalizing Turkey Tacos with Star
  Anise, 84–85
Tomatoes
 adding grated carrots to tomato sauce,
  184
 Alarmingly Good Low-Fat Chili,
  34–35
 Baked Eggs and Ham, 6
 Baked Meatballs with Zesty Marinara,
  86–87
 Breaded Zucchini with Marinara
  Dipping Sauce, 108–9★
 canned, cooking with, 90
 Chicken and Rice Hot Pot, 76–77
 Creamy Mexican Bean Dip with
  Whole Grain Tortilla Chips, 41
 French Tuna Salad, 62–63
 Good Lookin' Grilled Cheese, 57
 Light Lasagna Made with Turkey and
  Veggies, 54–55★
 Meatball Sandwiches, 88–89★
 Pigs in a Blanket, 90–91
 simple tomato sauce, preparing, 89
 Spicy Sloppy Joes with Carrot and
  Red Bell Pepper, 94–95
 Stuffed Peppers Cooked in Pepperoni-
  Flavored Tomato Sauce, 58–59
 Tantalizing Turkey Tacos with Star
  Anise, 84–85
Tortillas
 Creamy Mexican Bean Dip with
  Whole Grain Tortilla Chips, 41
 Garlicky Black Bean Soup, 30–31
 My Dad's Trim Chicken Enchiladas,
  67★
 Nachos Grande with Pickled Jalapeño
  Salsa, 42–43
Tuna
 French Tuna Salad, 62–63
 Mock Crab Cakes with Zucchini and
  Tuna, 64
 Rainbow Macaroni Salad with Tuna,
  60
Turkey
 adding to breakfast sandwich, 184
 Alarmingly Good Low-Fat Chili,
  34–35
 Baked Meatballs with Zesty Marinara,
  86–87
 cooking tip, 82
 flavoring, with herbs and spices, 82
 Good Lookin' Grilled Cheese, 57
 Light Lasagna Made with Turkey and
  Veggies, 54–55★

 Meatball Sandwiches, 88–89★
 Nachos Grande with Pickled Jalapeño
  Salsa, 42–43
 Pigs in a Blanket, 90–91
 Stuffed Peppers Cooked in Pepperoni-
  Flavored Tomato Sauce, 58–59
 Supermoist Turkey Burgers, 82–83
 Tantalizing Turkey Tacos with Star
  Anise, 84–85
Turkey bacon
 adding to salad dressing, 176
 Bacon, Egg, and Cheese Sandwich, 3
 Bacon Sausage Omelet with Onions
  and Peppers, 4–5
 Bacon Spinach Salad, 116
 Bacon-Wrapped Dates, 40
 benefits of, 3
 Broccoli Bacon Salad, 113
 Cut the Fat, Keep the Creamy Pasta
  Carbonara, 51
 Shrimp and Corn Chowder, 37★
 Twice-Baked Potatoes with Filling So
  Rich No One Will Know It's Low
  Fat, 104

USDA dietary recommendations, xxvii–
 xxviii

Vanilla
 Hot Fudge Sundae with Vanilla Bean
  Frozen Yogurt, 161
 Vanilla Bean "Ice Cream," 160
Vegetables. See also specific vegetables
 adding to chilis and soups, 35
 adding to frozen treats, 158
 adding to meals, xx, 13, 52, 57
 daily recommended servings, xxvii
 Four Food Groups Minestrone, 32–33
 grated, adding to recipes, xx, 13, 52
 Light Lasagna Made with Turkey and
  Veggies, 54–55★
 in quick meal ideas, 177–78
Vegetable slicers, 105
Vinegar, adding to baked goods, 150

Waffles
 adding cooked grains to, 152
 Maple Apple Waffles, 14–15
Walnuts
 adding to muffin recipe, 18

Apple Strudel with Walnut Crumble
  Topping, 148–49
 Banana Bread, 150–51
 My Granny's Cinnamon Coffee Cake
  the Skinny Way, 140–41
 omega-3 fatty acids in, xxi
 Slender Blondie Brownies with
  Walnuts, Chocolate Chips, and
  Prunes, 146–47★
 Zucchini Pancakes with Walnuts and
  Spice, 12–13
Water chestnuts
 Pork Lo Mein, Hold the Grease,
  92–93
Water intake, xxiv–xxv
Wheat germ
 adding to muffin recipe, 18
 Party Mix with Spiced Nuts and
  Whole Grain Cereal,
  46–47
White whole-wheat flour, about, 146

Yogurt
 Blueberry Cobbler with Yogurt
  Topping, 134–35
 Buttermilk Yogurt Dressing, 117
 Chocolate Breakfast Shake, 22
 Cut the Fat, Keep the Creamy Pasta
  Carbonara, 51
 Essential Smoothie, 23
 Frozen Coconut Yogurt, 159★
 Hot Fudge Sundae with Vanilla Bean
  Frozen Yogurt, 161
 Lemony Yogurt Muffins,
  18–19
 "Mayonnaise Is Not Your Enemy"
  Coleslaw, 112
 Party Dip Served with Whole Wheat
  Pita, 45
 Vanilla Bean "Ice Cream," 160

Zesters, 16
Zucchini
 Breaded Zucchini with Marinara
  Dipping Sauce, 108–9★
 Meatball Sandwiches, 88–89★
 Mock Crab Cakes with Zucchini and
  Tuna, 64
 Zucchini Bread for Breakfast, Too,
  152–53
 Zucchini Pancakes with Walnuts and
  Spice, 12–13